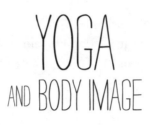

YOGA
AND BODY IMAGE

About the Authors

Melanie Klein, MA (Santa Monica, CA), is a writer, speaker, and Professor of Sociology and Women's Studies. As a body image advocate and proponent of media literacy education, she is also the cofounder of the Yoga and Body Image Coalition, on the advisory board for the Brave Girls Alliance, and the founder and co-coordinator of the LA chapter of Women, Action & the Media.

Anna Guest-Jelley, MA (Nashville, TN), is the founder of CurvyYoga .com, a training and inspiration portal for curvy yogis that has been featured in *The Washington Post, Yoga Journal, US News & World Report,* and *Yoga International,* among others.

MELANIE KLEIN & ANNA GUEST-JELLEY

YOGA
AND BODY IMAGE

25 Personal Stories

About Beauty, Bravery

& Loving Your Body

Llewellyn Publications
Woodbury, Minnesota

FIRST EDITION
First Printing, 2014

Cover design by Kevin R. Brown
Cover photo: Sarit Z. Rogers / Sarit Photography; Model: Courtney Sauls

Llewellyn Publications is a registered trademark of Llewellyn Worldwide Ltd.

Library of Congress Cataloging-in-Publication Data

Klein, Melanie, 1972–
   Yoga and body image : 25 personal stories about beauty, bravery & loving your body /
by Melanie Klein, Anna Guest-Jelley. — First Edition.
      pages cm
   ISBN 978-0-7387-3982-3
1. Yoga—Psychological aspects. 2. Yoga--Social aspects. 3. Body image. 4. Yogis—Biography. I. Guest-Jelley, Anna. II. Title.
   RA781.67.K54 2014
   613.7'046—dc23
                                  2014028269

Llewellyn Worldwide Ltd. does not participate in, endorse, or have any authority or responsibility concerning private business transactions between our authors and the public.
   All mail addressed to the author is forwarded, but the publisher cannot, unless specifi-cally instructed by the author, give out an address or phone number.
   Any Internet references contained in this work are current at publication time, but the publisher cannot guarantee that a specific location will continue to be maintained. Please refer to the publisher's website for links to authors' websites and other sources.
   Cover model(s) used for illustrative purposes only and may not endorse or represent the book's subject matter.

Llewellyn Publications
A Division of Llewellyn Worldwide Ltd.
2143 Wooddale Drive
Woodbury, MN 55125-2989
www.llewellyn.com

Printed in the United States of America

Contents

PART FIVE: GENDER AND SEXUALITY - 211

WHY YOGA AND BODY IMAGE

Melanie Klein

I first met my coeditor, Anna Guest-Jelley, in 2010. I was introduced to her work through her blog post "Welcoming the Curvy Yogini," which was about how to make space for bigger-bodied students in yoga. I was instantly enthralled. Not only did Anna's words and experience speak to me, but I was taken by her bio wherein she described herself as "an advocate for women's rights by day, a yoga teacher by night." Given my experience as a sociology and women's studies professor paired with my activist work and a yoga practice reaching back to the mid-nineties, I knew I had stumbled upon a kindred spirit. I was compelled to collaborate with her.

As an academic with a background and continued interest in a variety of healing modalities, I often felt out of place in both worlds. I had been regularly practicing yoga since 1996, became a certified massage therapist in 2000 through the Institute of Psycho-Structural Balancing, completed my advanced training as a Thai Yoga Therapy practitioner with Saul David Raye in 2001, took a yoga teacher training with Ganga White and Tracy Rich at the White Lotus Foundation in 2002, and had developed a consistent meditation practice after two ten-day Vipassana meditation retreats as taught by S. N. Goenka. During all this, though, it often appeared my rigorous academic training and critical thinking skills were seen as a deterrent or hindrance in this realm. Based on several experiences writing for the yoga community, it became evident to me that critical thinking was not necessarily welcomed or encouraged.

Simultaneously, I was actively involved in feminist politics, social justice movements, media literacy education, advocacy work, and the completion of two degrees in sociology with an emphasis on the intersection of gender, race, and class. To many in those arenas, yoga, meditation, and holistic healing seemed new-agey, trivial, and empty navel-gazing. In fact, my academic mentors could never figure out what my yoga practice had to do with my educational and professional goals.

But the connections between my sociological imagination, feminist consciousness, and advocacy work with yoga have always been obvious to me—they all represent opportunities to raise our consciousness, take a holistic perspective on our individual problems, become our best selves, and create a more equitable and balanced world.

Blended Worlds

I began merging these backgrounds and areas of interest by applying my sociological imagination to a newly burgeoning yoga culture. In 2004 and 2005, I presented on yoga, popular culture, and commodification at four different academic conferences: "The McDonaldization and Commodification of Yoga: Standing at the Intersection of Spiritual Tradition and Consumer Culture" at the Pacific Sociological Association, "Consuming Spirituality and Spiritual Consuming: Capitalizing on Yoga" at the California Sociological Association, "McYoga: The Spiritual Diet for a Consumer America" at the Far West Popular Culture and American Culture Association, and "Yoga and Popular Culture" at the California Sociological Association. Anna was the first person I had come across who shared a similar background. She had earned several degrees and had a professional background in which she worked as an English professor, ran a renowned domestic violence prevention program, comanaged a university women's center, published papers, and created workshops and coordinated community programs on universal health care, reproductive rights, adult literacy, wellness, and emotional resilience. When it came to eating disorders, abuse, self-neglect, and anxiety—you name it, Anna had written the curriculum, xeroxed the worksheets, and hung the "Welcome" sign on the door.

I needed to connect with this woman. In my gut, I knew we were destined to collaborate and merge our efforts, talents, and skills into a broader conversation that bridged these seemingly disparate worlds. These two spheres of influence had so much to teach each other, and that marriage would only benefit and, hopefully, connect the members of each population.

Anna and I eventually had our first phone conversation in the spring of 2011 and the synergy was immediately palpable. We realized that a joint endeavor was undeniable. After a few months of percolating, we realized it only made sense to collaborate on a book focusing on yoga and body image.

Anna and I have not only each maintained a consistent yoga and meditation practice since the mid-nineties, but we are actively engaged with and play an active role in the larger yoga community. While we write for a variety of platforms, much of our writing is specifically published by publications advocating mind/body wellness. In this vein, Anna and I are among the pioneers and leaders who have opened a line of inquiry exploring the connection between yoga and body image. While conversations about yoga and body image have increased in the blogosphere in the last few years, *Yoga from the Inside Out: Making Peace with Your Body Through Yoga* by Christina Sell, *May I Be Happy: A Memoir of Love, Yoga, and Changing My Mind* by Cyndi Lee, my chapter exploring the connection between feminism, pop culture, body image, and yoga in *21st Century Yoga: Culture, Politics and Practice* (eds. Carol Horton and Roseanne Harvey), and *Curvy Voices*, Anna's collection of stories about yoga and body acceptance, are among the first book publications *specifically* exploring yoga and body image in contemporary yoga culture in the new millennium.

In addition to writing and shaping conversations within the yoga community, we have both created and facilitated workshops on wellness, yoga, and body image. I am approached more and more often about delivering speeches that specifically address the interplay between yoga, body image, and pop culture for body image summits, conferences aimed at empowering girls and women, as well as talks and workshops for Women's History

Month, Love Your Body Week, and the National Eating Disorders Association's annual Eating Disorder Awareness Week. Anna has been teaching yoga classes that create space for women of all sizes to develop a yoga practice. She has also created curriculum to train yoga teachers to be mindful of body image issues and differences in size, thereby producing teachers who have the tools, techniques, and language to guide and teach curvy students. Her Curvy Yoga classes are now being taught in multiple countries and across the United States.

How This Book Came to Be

We decided on this topic because it's something we're both passionate about and our work over the years reflects that interest. We are both staunch body image advocates with a long history of advocacy work, curriculum development, and research combining the insight and analysis developed in academia, media literacy training, social activism, our yogic background along with a variety of other healing modalities, and our life experiences.

We are committed to not only creating dialogue about the ways in which self-love may be cultivated (and why that's a necessary step in maximizing our own life experience thereby allowing us to participate and contribute more fully in the larger culture), but offering yoga as a tangible tool that can make that happen—if one consistently practices with a particular mindset and level of consciousness.

It's not enough to encourage people to love their bodies through positive slogans and affirmations, such as "Love your body!" If people knew how, they would! We think it's crucial in our body-focused culture that perpetuates a one-size-does-NOT-fit-all standard of beauty to provide a practice that can help facilitate that acceptance and self-love. But we also wanted to explore the intersection of yoga and body image because it's an area we don't see discussed often enough in the yoga community. Though they are often so focused on the body itself, yoga classes and conversations rarely include the topic of how we *feel* about our body and how yoga affects our body image and vice versa.

And to us, that is a major gap in the conversation—not only how individuals' body image can benefit from yoga, but also how yoga has a complicated place in the conversation about body image, both contributing to negative perceptions via media stereotypes of the "yoga body" and contributing to positive change when the practice is focused on connection with one's body, exactly as it is today.

The primary focus of this book is on the transformative benefits of a yoga *practice* on the body-mind. But the conversation would not be complete without mentioning the *culture* of yoga that has sprung up, for better or worse, in the last decade along with the yoga *industry*. It is possible to be critical and aware of the changes in the culture while hailing the many positive benefits the practice offers. In fact, without turning a critical eye to the images and ideas that influence our body image, we believe it is near impossible to create any substantial change. We have to work on the micro and the macro level at the same time.

While Anna and I could have written a book on yoga and body image based on our own powerful experiences of transformation as a result of a regular practice, we were and are fiercely committed to bringing together a diverse collection of voices that span across the spectrum of human experience.

Yoga and Body Image

Body image refers to an ideal image of one's body, an image that is intellectual and subjective. This psychological image of one's body is shaped from a lifetime of observations, experiences, and reactions from others, such as family members, peers, and the media. Race and ethnicity, sexual orientation, sex, gender identity, size, age, class, and physical ability all play significant roles in the formation of one's body image. And, too often, the reflection we see in the mirror is a grossly distorted image of ourselves influenced by our experiences, interpretations, and expectations. As a result, much of our dissatisfaction (and disappointment) with our bodies and compromised self-esteem is a result of an image not rooted in reality but grounded in an illusion.

Yoga practitioners and those plagued by distorted body image issues do not come in a uniform mold. We wanted to reach readers of different backgrounds, casting a wide net and allowing people to draw inspiration from at least one contributor's body image journey and how their yoga practice facilitated that transformation. We feel yoga and the potential healing benefits are for every body. No body should be excluded from having access to the practice. We believe in the power of the practice and its ability to change lives and communities for the better.

Though no anthology can be completely representative of every community, we feel that our efforts to be inclusive are evident. While the experiences and journeys of our contributors often run parallel to and complement one another, each is unique in exploring a particular sense of self and body.

In Part One, Linda Sparrowe, Dr. Sara Gottfried, Marianne Elliott, Dr. Melody Moore, and my coeditor Anna open the book by talking about the ways in which yoga allows us to expand our options and our perspectives. Yoga is truly about "Making Choices and Creating Change." In fact, Anna and I feel that this is at the heart of a yoga practice—the potential to create profound changes. Yoga develops our ability to listen and it raises our consciousness to become more present in each moment of our lives.

In Part Two, Vytas Baskauskas, Dianne Bondy, Carrie Barrepski, Teo Drake, and Joni Yung share their experience of existing "On the Margins"—feeling out of place and being "the other" in some capacity, being excluded from adolescent peer culture, or not conforming to the conventional able-bodied, Eurocentric, size-0 beauty ideal, or the expectation of the "yoga body." Often that feeling of marginalization has included yoga culture itself. But, in the end, each individual moves to a place of integration—and the practice plays, and continues to play, a key role in coming to a space of wholeness. As Vytas readily admits, it's a work in progress, a daily practice of self-love and acceptance along with shifting one's perspective.

In Part Three, I explore "Culture and Media" along with Rolf Gates, Nita Rubio, Seane Corn, Chelsea Jackson, and Alanis Morissette. Not only do we examine the role of mainstream culture and the mass media in framing our expectations of ideal masculinity and femininity, several of us examine the downside to yoga culture and the ways in which it replicates idealized and impossible images of beauty. We discuss the ways in which a yoga practice can diminish this cultural noise and argue that culture is what we make it. We can create change that leads to a beauty standard that fits everyone.

In Part Four, "Parenting and Children," Kate McIntyre Clere, Claire Mysko, Dr. Dawn M. Dalili, and Shana Meyerson tackle consumer culture, the salacious and unforgiving tabloid industry, and advertising, as well as distorted body images, eating disorders, and the challenge to raise healthy and confident children in an often toxic media culture while simultaneously struggling with their own self-esteem. They write about the pressures of bump-watch, the joy of creation, and the value of teaching yoga to children, many of whom have already begun to learn to hate their bodies.

In Part Five, "Gender and Sexuality," Rosie Molinary, Dr. Kerrie Kauer, Bryan Kest, Ryan McGraw, and Dr. Audrey Bilger examine sexual orientation, sex, and the gendered body as related to yoga. As a group, they urge us to consider the myriad ways that yoga can transform the relationship to one's body as a reflection of one's gender identity and sexual orientation. From culturally sanctioned notions of violent masculinity and the "proper" way to be a "real" man to sexualization, sexism, heterosexism, and homophobia, the yoga practice provides peace, solace, and healing for the contributors in this section.

As a whole, whether their bodily disassociation was a result of objectification, race, class, sex, sexual orientation, gender identity, disability, size, shape, or an "outsider" status, yoga provided the opportunity for this collection of writers to know and love themselves in an authentic and extraordinary new way.

What Yoga Can Do

Unlike many of the solutions offered in a culture rooted in instant gratification, yoga will not transform our body image overnight. As Anna reminds us in the conclusion, creating a healthy relationship to self and healing a fractured body image is a work in progress, like anything else meaningful and long lasting.

Similarly, Anna encourages us to utilize yoga as a tool in conjunction with others that may be uniquely helpful to us. For some that may mean seeking the advice of a doctor, therapist, or nutritionist in tandem with our practice. For me, my feminist consciousness and academic training provided the intellectual grounding that supported the self-inquiry and spiritual growth that resulted from my yoga practice. For Anna, the support of therapy, meditation, feminist activism, and body-positive yoga friends helped her learn to accept and love her body. And for just about everyone, it means finding solace and support in a community of like-minded individuals.

Our intention is to inspire people who have an interest in developing a practice to begin exploring their options, especially those who thought yoga wasn't for them. We also want current practitioners to begin or expand inquiry into how yoga and body image intersect in their communities.

A yoga practice can and should be available to everyone and *every* body. Begin by trying out different teachers and classes in person or explore the ever-increasing range of options online or on DVD. Explore and experiment with teachers, classes, and styles until you find the practice that speaks to you and encourages you to be gentle, kind, and compassionate with your body.

We also want yoga teachers to begin cultivating healthy dialogue in class that allows the yoga practice to nurture students in a noncompetitive environment by focusing on the quality of mind, not the aesthetics of the pose or the body in the pose. You don't have to have a perfect body image or all the answers to begin creating this space in class. Yoga teachers are human too, and they have to do the work just like everyone else.

Let's celebrate our humanity in all its diversity—the shapes, sizes, abilities, ages, and colors that make the human race special. Let's celebrate our bodies, open our hearts, and grow our spirits in this practice. Let's raise our consciousness and our awareness. Because of its focus on union (since that's the definition!), yoga is uniquely situated to facilitate this process. When we engage in it, we're able to move past the clutter, learn how to listen, and make authentic choices about how we see ourselves and move through the world.

PART ONE

Making Choices and Creating Change

We chose to start the book with this section because of how the authors frame the question, problem, and opportunity inherent in yoga as a tool for working with body image. As it's practiced in the West today, yoga has the possibility of becoming a way into a deeper, more positive relationship with one's body—and it also has the possibility of reinscribing limiting beauty and body norms.

Linda Sparrowe starts us off with just that question: How can yoga help—or hinder—one's relationship with their body? Through insight and conversation with others, she guides us through an exploration of how yoga is showing up currently in the context of yoga and body image.

Next, Dr. Sara Gottfried takes us into the practical realm of yoga and how it's much more than a workout, as it's often portrayed. From her perspective as a Harvard-educated physician, she leads us through the many ways that yoga can support people, both in their body and in their relationship with it.

From there, Marianne Elliott shares her story of how shame showed up on her yoga mat and what she did to shift it. Through the lens of this story, she leaves us with a call to action for how yoga can be a practice of kindness, first and foremost to ourselves.

Next, Dr. Melody Moore talks about the feeling she had growing up of not being or doing enough—and how that ever-raised bar of expectations showed up in her relationship with her body. She shares how yoga was a way out and a door into her current work, supporting people around disordered eating and body image.

Finally, Anna Guest-Jelley shares one of her major life aha moments: when it dawned on her that maybe the reason she didn't feel comfortable practicing yoga in a bigger body wasn't because of her body, but rather because of how yoga was often taught to one particular body type—and how yoga has the potential to welcome people of all shapes and sizes.

COMING HOME TO THE BODY: CAN YOGA HELP OR HINDER?

Linda Sparrowe

Years ago, as part of a special promotion, a few of us donned Capezio outfits that left little to the imagination, performed 15-minute yoga demonstrations in the fitness section of Macy's, and then spoke to a small band of curious onlookers about the benefits of what we kept calling "this amazing practice." At the end of the talk, a woman came up to me, with two of her friends in tow, and said, "So, what do you think? Twenty? Maybe thirty?" I had no idea what she meant. "Twenty, maybe thirty what?" I asked. *"Pounds,"* she said. "How many pounds do I need to lose before I sign up for yoga?" When I told her that no one had to lose anything to go to a yoga class, the woman looked at me and said, "Yeah, right. I'm going to put clothes like yours over thighs like mine and walk into a room full of beautiful bodies. Why? So I can feel worse about myself? No, thanks." Her friends nodded knowingly and nothing we said could convince them otherwise.

Bastardizing the Practice

These ladies had a point. Why indeed? Although that conversation took place many years ago, and I haven't been in a body-hugging Capezio outfit since, I still think of them from time to time and wonder if they ever set foot in a yoga class. I like to think they did and that they enjoyed it. I certainly want to believe that yoga offers a more conscious and inclusive experience than it did back then, but I'm not sure it does. Yoga has long evolved to meet the needs of the culture it serves, and unfortunately it's currently serving a culture that equates thin and young with healthy and perfect. As a result, many yoga classes overemphasize the physical and attract students who already have lithe, athletic bodies. So, not surprisingly, those who don't fit that narrow description feel left out. As another of the women wondered, how would doing 60 to 90 minutes of stretchy, bendy, sweaty yoga poses with a bunch of skinny, flexible, young women make her feel any better about her self-described plump, stiff, old body?

How indeed? Now that I'm inching into my 60s, I get it. Just walking into most yoga classes can have a demoralizing effect on anyone who feels self-conscious or ashamed of their body (at last count, at least 90 percent of women polled). But I can't honestly fault yoga completely, nor do I mean to suggest that all contemporary yoga teachers are interchangeable with aerobics instructors. But the lack of authentic practice in some classes keeps yoga confined to the realm of the get-thin-quick solutions. The sages of old never meant for *asana*—the postures or poses in yoga—to represent the whole of this spiritual path. But too often they do. And when we practice *asana* devoid of any meditative aspect, our focus gets stuck on the physical body—usually on those parts we hate—and we lose connection with our breath, our intuition, and our deeper selves. This "bastardization of yoga," a phrase coined by Melody Moore, PhD, a clinical psychologist in Dallas specializing in treating women with eating disorders, keeps us in a state of being "not enough" and tethered to whatever limitations we deem unacceptable.

Of course, those limitations can be anything. While the majority of women believe they are too fat, others hate looking too old, being too stiff or weak or ugly or … a thousand different "too this or not enough that." Moore reminded me that teachers have this amazing opportunity to create a safe space for their students to let go of such beliefs. Indeed, as Donna Farhi, a New Zealand–based author and yoga teacher, says, "It is through the teacher's search for and commitment to her own authenticity that a student gains permission for her innate being to shine forth."

Moving from Wholeness

Unfortunately, those yoga teachers whose authentic teaching helps others "shine forth" can sometimes get caught up in Western culture's obsession with (and definition of) physical perfection themselves. Not long ago a friend of mine wrote me, upset that a "famous teacher" whose workshop she had signed up for had misrepresented herself by posting a photo that was at least a couple decades old. If we are really yogis, she said, "we shouldn't be afraid that someone won't come to our workshop because we're not 25 and a size 0." She found the teacher's deception appalling and inherently shaming of the aging process for women. When yoga teachers are ashamed of their aging bodies, they send a pretty powerful message to their students that says being young, thin, and hip are all that matters. Instead, they need to present themselves fully—wrinkles, gray hair, laugh lines, and all—and step into exactly who they are: wise and beautiful. I do see how difficult that is in a world where youthful beauty trumps all; to do that, we all need courage, strength, and good role models.

So how do we—students *and* teachers—move beyond this fixation with the physical body to a place where we can feel better about ourselves? First of all, we need to stop thinking of yoga as something that will make us thinner, younger, and richer. We need to then embrace *asana* as part of a deeper practice that includes how we treat ourselves and others (the *yamas* and *niyamas*), breathing techniques (*pranayama*), sensory withdrawal (*pratyahara*), concentration (*dharana*), meditation (*dhyana*), and liberation (*samadhi*). Once that happens, we can experience yoga's benefits on every level of our being—physical, mental, emotional, and spiritual—and yoga can become a powerful antidote to self-loathing.

I'm not suggesting, of course, that yoga should exclude the physical body and go directly to our more spiritual or ethereal side. Yoga, after all, is a *body-based* practice, and we can never heal our wounded self-image if we shun the body. We have to agree to be there, get to know ourselves on a musculoskeletal and cellular level. Not always easy, but if you approach yoga with a sense of self-compassion and curiosity, you may find that nothing quite compares to feeling the steadiness of your feet on the floor, knowing that those thighs you've hated all your life are actually the perfect size, shape, and strength to hold you up. Those arms that jiggle back at you when you look in the mirror hold you up in a handstand, extend so beautifully in Warrior pose, or allow you to press back into an almost comfortable Downward-Facing Dog for five breaths. For that moment, during those breaths, your relationship with your body changes and your mind forgets its litany of judgmental complaints. Those individual body parts remain the same—they probably still jiggle, shake, and sag—but your experience of them radically changes. Whatever judgments you habitually heap on your body fall away and you move from a sense of wholeness.

Yoga brings the mind and body together in a common goal: to guide us inward and reconnect us to our true nature, our innate goodness. That true nature includes all parts of us—not just the ones we like. The breath, acting as a bridge between the body and mind, creates a partnership that supports our ability to love ourselves and let go of what no longer serves us. In this way, yoga ultimately transforms us. Not in the way a diet plan or exercise program does—yoga doesn't promise to whittle down the size of your thighs or smooth out your wrinkles. But it can radically change your relationship to those thighs or stop you from obsessing about your neck. In order for that to happen, however, you need to spend some time learning how to appreciate the body you have. The best way I know to do that? Step onto the yoga mat.

Healing the Rift

If you had a falling out with a close friend and wanted to reconcile, how would you do that? Would you spend your time going over all of the horrible things she said to you, reviewing all of her bad qualities in great detail? Probably not. More than likely you would think a little wistfully about the good times you shared, all the times she was there for you, and all the things that made you love her in the first place. In order to patch things up, you would need to see her, talk with her, and maybe renew your commitment to be a kinder, more attentive friend.

Can you do that with your own body? Can you approach it as lovingly as you would your own best friend, regardless of how estranged that relationship had become? Can you use your yoga practice to be a kinder friend—to yourself? Much like a damaged friendship, the more you abuse your body or ignore its needs, the more you suffer. Corrine Wainer, director of YoGirls, an after-school yoga literacy and wellness program in New York City, says yoga helped her become friends with her severely dislocated shoulder recently. While everyone else in class was in Downward-Facing Dog, Corrine had to do Plank pose, and lifting her arms in Warrior I was completely out of the question. She started to feel a little emotional, but realized that by moving slowly and respectfully—and not comparing herself to anyone else—she was honoring what her body needed at that moment to heal.

Yoga allowed Corrine to explore her body from the inside out—not from a preconceived notion of what it should be able to do. She worked with her shoulder tenderly, much like she would with a friend in pain, noticing how it responded to certain movements and discovering what it needed to feel better and ultimately get stronger.

Silencing the Self-Critic

Showing up for your body like Corrine did takes a lot of willpower. Some days will definitely be easier than others. I try to approach my practice from a place of compassionate self-inquiry (what yoga calls *svadhyaya*), bringing my mind into my body and letting go of outside stimulation. When that happens, I don't think about my age or the image that stares back at me in the mirror. On my mat, I allow my breath to move me from pose to pose and I feel strong and connected and at peace. But on those days when I can't seem to do an arm balance to save my life or when I have to come out of a standing pose before everyone else? I feel like I've lost my way, and my mind goes right back to its old self-deprecating ways: How can I possibly call myself a yoga teacher when I can't even do yoga? Am I a sham? And whose tight hip flexors are these anyway? Obviously, switching up a poor self-image takes more than just willpower or hours of vinyasa practice. It takes loving kindness, patience, generosity, and self-reflection *without judgment*—what Swami Kripalu called the highest form of spiritual practice.

The issues we have with our bodies run deep. In fact, therapists like to say that those issues live in our tissues. The trauma we've experienced, the anger or hurt we stuff down, can manifest as anything from a clenched jaw, painful hip, or tight neck muscles to a persistent sense of sadness or free-floating anxiety. If we don't figure out a way to release our negative emotions, the attendant physical pains could escalate to more serious problems such as self-destructive behaviors (addictions, eating disorders), panic attacks, metabolic syndrome, digestive disorders, or even autoimmune diseases.

To release all that tension in the body, we need to calm the mind. When the mind stops reacting and comes to a place of stillness, the body can too. And of course, as researchers have known for a long time, a restful body and a calm mind reduce stress, which lowers cortisol (stress hormone) levels, balances the nervous system, and heals or prevents stress-related illnesses. Incorporating meditation and *pratyahara* into your *asana* practice will help you tune out external distractions that cause the mind to spin out of control and then turn inward. Noticing, softening, and releasing any pain or agitation will allow you to experience a deep-seated sense of calm acceptance. This happened to my friend Robin, which came as a complete surprise to her.

After suffering through years of bulimia as a young woman, Robin had a tenuous relationship, at best, with her body. But she didn't come to yoga with any idea of changing that. Her motivation was strictly physical. She needed to rehab after knee surgery and her doctor insisted she try yoga. "My leg muscles had atrophied as a result of the surgery," she said. "I had no choice but to embrace my limitations since the whole reason I began yoga was to increase my leg's strength and agility." But a funny thing happened on the way to a stronger leg. Once she accepted that she couldn't get her knee to the floor in a seated pose and that her leg wobbled in Warrior pose, she found herself accepting other limitations and imperfections. A few months later, she remembered, "I startled myself when I looked in the mirror while getting dressed and

thought, 'Hey, I look pretty darn good.' I couldn't remember *ever* thinking that before, certainly not with any conviction."

As Robin discovered, yoga puts us in touch with our "pretty darn
good" self and helps us see that we actually have a pretty darn *perfect*
self, even with an atrophied leg, a separated shoulder, 30 extra pounds,
or a multitude of laugh lines. That can only happen, however, when we
engage the mind and the heart and stop obsessing about what we see in
the mirror.

Engaging the Mind

Linking the physical practice of *asana* to the mental/emotional realm
through *pranayama*, *pratyahara*, and meditation is critical to our healing.
While a more mindful yoga practice won't necessarily get rid of your
self-critic, it can point out and even temper the incessant negative chatter that your mind often defaults to. Conscious breathing and mindful
awareness move the mind away from external judgments and deeper
into the body. I know when I become disconnected to my breath or
when my mind goes on one of its judgmental tangents, my body feels
abandoned and gets off kilter. Working with the breath, connecting it
to *asana* or simply sitting in meditation, allows me to pause often and
listen deeply. In those pauses between the inhale and exhale (especially
the pause right after the exhale), sometimes everything coalesces, and in
that still moment of acceptance, all negativity melts away.

When I am confronted with thoughts and feelings that play out like
a broken record, I have to stop, come back to my body—moving my
awareness into my feet or exhaling into my tight hip—and recommit
to my basic goodness. This fresh start helps me to replace any blame or
shame I feel with a nonjudgmental "isn't that interesting" mantra.

Even substituting more loving language for your standard invective
will make a big difference in how you approach your body and, in turn,
how it responds to your care. Simply replacing the thought "I hate my
left hip. It's always so tight. It never does what I want it to" with "I need
to give my tight left hip a little more loving attention today. It doesn't
seem very happy right now" makes your body feel love instead of con-
tempt. Switching out negativity for curiosity allows you to silence the

inner critic more often and choose self-love instead. If you approach yoga with the intention of learning more about yourself—instead of *changing* more of yourself—you'll come to trust your own abilities and discover what's truly best for you.

Embracing the Love

Recently someone sent me an ad campaign from a soap product. Its tag line read: *When did you stop thinking you were beautiful?* During the campaign, when faced with getting their picture taken, grown women hid from the camera and young girls clamored to steal the spotlight. That certainly gave me pause. When indeed? When do we stop thinking we're beautiful? Could it be when we opt to look outside ourselves for validation, comparing ourselves to someone else's attributes, someone else's accomplishments, and forget to notice our own? When we lose connection to the deepest part of ourselves, we lose sight of our basic goodness and our inner (and outer) beauty.

So how do we get that connection back? By practicing diligently, showing up for ourselves no matter what—like a good friend does—and letting go of destructive thoughts and behaviors that keep us from happiness. In other words, we need to work hard, listen deeply, and let compassion guide our choices. When a thought surfaces during class (or in your everyday life), ask yourself, "Is this kind? Does this support my intention to love myself?" If not, let it go.

This shift doesn't happen overnight. I get a little nervous sometimes when I hear teachers tell their students that yoga will radically transform them. I don't want people to think of yoga as the "big fix" in their lives. What if you don't feel a shift at first? Does that make you even more of a loser than you think you are? No. Sometimes that shift is subtle. Sometimes a single exhale relieves you of your usual negative thoughts. That's actually a huge shift, but when you've spent a lifetime in a body you despise, you may not even notice it. Even if you do, those negative thoughts (or others) may resurface and you'll have to replace them with more loving ones again and again.

That's why they call yoga a *practice*. The more you experience these exquisite moments of self-love and the more you dwell in delight, the more your negative actions, thoughts, and feelings will begin to dissipate. And as they do, you may find what is left is the body you fell in love with many years ago and you've come back home.

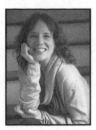

Linda Sparrowe is the author of several books on yoga and the former editor of both *Yoga International* and *Yoga Journal*. She teaches trauma-sensitive yoga as a way for women to come back home to their bodies and joyfully awaken to their true nature. www.lindasparrowe.com
Author photo by Sarah Forbes Keough.

YOGA IS MORE THAN JUST A WORKOUT

Dr. Sara Gottfried

I can hardly think of a woman I know who doesn't complain about a muffin top, or wrinkles, or the restricted menu of her latest fad diet (one that is almost guaranteed to fail). Women have a neurotic preoccupation with a distorted body image, weight, and fatness. I'm one of those women, perpetually recovering from my obsession with weight.

Unfortunately, few of us are armed with the tools and resources we need to reclaim the body we want, the corresponding body image, and the self-confidence we need to live a long life of contentment and vitality. I want to change that. My goal is to change the conversation about weight and body image, and to get us to a *wabi-sabi* way of looking at the female form. Yoga is one of the most powerful vehicles to help us view the world through the lens of wabi-sabi. I'm not the first to point this out—the latest way to approach the healing of your body and body image also happens to be one of the oldest ways.

Enter Wabi-Sabi

Most simply, wabi-sabi is the Japanese art of finding beauty and wisdom in imperfection, such as a lovely tea bowl with cracks and chips that has aged uniquely. We are all imperfect and flawed, and there is tremendous beauty in not just accepting this as true but reveling in and honoring the imperfection.

Wabi-sabi is an antidote to the false ideal of the perfect female form.

Anyone, male or female, living in today's media-saturated world is bombarded with images of bodily perfection and what I consider to be the glorified ideal of the anorexic adolescent. Online ads feature stick-thin models (most of whom are genetic outliers); e-mail newsletters tout the latest celebrity diets; and commercials and movies showcase the willowy, the tan, and the glossy-haired. Unfortunately, instead of a society focused on attaining vibrant health and longevity, we've turned into a community of people obsessed with looking thin and young, at any cost.

How Perfection Harms Us

This epidemic of dissatisfied women and negative body image reveals itself in several ways.

Stress

The pressure to look a certain way only adds to the already-frazzled nerves and busy schedules of most modern women. Tanning treatments, gym sessions, Botox, buying the right skinny jeans … who has the time? In addition, our dogged pursuit of perfect beauty, often bordering on self-violence, raises cortisol, the main stress hormone.

Cortisol levels are at a record high level, and hormonal imbalances are, as a result, rampant. This is not just theoretical: research from the lab of Nobel Prize laureate Elizabeth Blackburn at the University of California at San Francisco shows that premenopausal women with high perceived stress age ten years faster than women with normal levels of stress. She documented the accelerated aging by measuring the telomeres, the caps on chromosomes that track your biological aging as opposed to your chronological aging, in stressed women versus controls.

Lack of Body Awareness

Instead of looking inward and listening to what our bodies need (more sleep, vitamin D, maybe some acupuncture), we follow what advertising tells us to do, wear, or consume. Instead of cultivating healthy lifestyle habits, we're constantly on the hunt for the magical pill that will solve all our problems. A lifestyle of cubicles, television, and general escapism means we no longer know our bodies.

Toxic Lifestyle

What many people don't realize is that a lifestyle that follows the suggestions of our current society is one that does the human body few favors. Cosmetics, processed foods, and synthetic textiles actually accelerate the aging process, the very problem they're supposed to solve!

We face a silent epidemic of overwhelm—we're cranky, fat, and have no sex drive because stress has hijacked our hormone balance. Most women run from task to task and don't realize how the main stress hormone (cortisol) is depleting the happy brain chemicals such as serotonin and dopamine, pulling your other hormones offline, accelerating the aging process, and setting you up for memory problems and perhaps Alzheimer's disease. Yet cortisol is a completely tangible hormone that you can manage like you would train a puppy or track your 401K.

Fear of Fatness

While most of us don't have a diagnosable "eating disorder," far too many people suffer from distorted body image. For lack of a scientific name, I like to call it Fear of Fatness (FOF), based on a wonderful essay by Jungian analyst Anne Ulenov. As a doctor board-certified in everything that can go wrong in the female body, I would apply this label to nearly every woman who walks through the front door of my practice. Once we start to review her pain points, it comes out: the eagle eye on daily weight changes, the angsty depression after "eating too much," the obsessively targeted exercise plans, the endless strategies to get back to the pre-pregnancy weight.

And I can relate. I'm one of the 90 percent of women who are dissatisfied with their bodies, constantly thinking about my weight and how my body looks on an hour-to-hour basis. Sadly, my perceived appearance can dictate my mood for the day. I'm sure I'm squandering far too much of my neuronal activity and energy bio-hacking my food plan, exercise, and lean body mass. For myself and the millions of people like me, it's not anorexia or bulimia, or psychosis exactly, but rather, it's "normal" for a female in this body-obsessed culture.

As a physician and scientist, the next question I ask is: Why? While cultural conditioning is certainly a factor, can I really blame the media for all these body image issues? No, I blame my tenuous connection to a deeper spiritual core. It's easier to focus on my distorted body image than on the true work that needs to be done on my inner self. The truth is that radical acceptance and cultivation of secular spiritual connection require a dedicated effort. And that takes a lot more time and effort than the South Beach Diet.

The wonderful news is that there *is* a solution to this disconnect. It isn't expensive, anyone can do it, and it's scientifically proven to address the issues I outlined above.

I'm talking yoga, my friends.

How Yoga Changed My Path

When I was in my 30s, I was working hard. I won't tell you that I was working too hard, but I was working without sufficient balance. My day job was as a doctor at a health maintenance organization (HMO), which I regard as my years in McMedicine. It meant seeing dozens of patients every day in assembly-line fashion, never stopping for a lunch break, and squeezing extra-extra hours of paperwork into the week whenever possible. I was often stressed out, angry, and resentful.

I was 25 pounds overweight and thought PMS stood for "Pass My Shotgun." I preferred a glass of wine to sex with my husband, didn't spend enough time with my girlfriends, was chronically low in oxytocin (the hormone of love, bonding, and social affiliation), and I can tell you that many modern women (and men) feel this way. I had never been unhealthier in my life.

And then I found yoga. Rather, I rediscovered yoga, because it was in my genes. Yoga had been part of my world before, but it took some serious overwhelm before I embraced it. Turns out, it was the optimal prescription for my stressed-out life.

Mud: Miracle Great-Granny

Growing up, I had an eccentric great-grandmother nicknamed Mud (my grandfather couldn't pronounce the full German word for "mother" and the name stuck). Mud was a whole-foodist. She never touched alcohol ("I love wine, but it doesn't love me"), she slept on a board ("good for the posture, my dear"), and she was a dedicated yogi decades before it was fashionable. She looked far younger than her peers, outlived four husbands, and rocked a vigorous, joyful life until she died peacefully in her sleep at age 97. Mud planted the seed early on in my mind that optimal health could be achieved through lifestyle and exercise, and often without pharmaceuticals.

Vitamin Y

When I started researching natural strategies for how to solve my stress, my weight gain, and my feelings of "meh," a world of hormone imbalances (and their amazingly simple preventive strategies) opened up before me. The most effective treatment that I found is an absolute powerhouse when it comes to reducing stress, losing weight, revving up metabolism, and increasing longevity. Yep: yoga.

I didn't just adopt a regular yoga practice—I became a certified yoga teacher and now share yoga's health benefits with anyone who will listen (we teach what we most need to learn). Luckily, when the yoga talk is backed by hard scientific data, you can hold the attention of even the most cynical doctors and patients.

It's not fair, but it's a fact: women are much more vulnerable to hormonal imbalance than men. Hormonal problems are the top reason I find for accelerated aging. Hormones are chemical messengers, like snail-mail in the body. They influence behavior, emotion, brain chemicals, the immune system, and how you turn food into fuel. When your hormones are in balance, neither too high nor too low, you look and feel your best. But when they are imbalanced, they become the mean girls in high school, making your life miserable. You can feel lethargic, irritable, weepy, grumpy, unappreciated, anxious, and depressed. Yoga is one of the most reliable ways to balance your hormones (especially their ringleader, cortisol), but it brings to the table a whole host of rejuvenating, life-extending benefits. The following are nine unexpected ways yoga improves body image and the innate intelligence of your body.

1. Yoga Lowers Stress (and Cortisol)

After decades of balancing the hormones of thousands of women, I can confidently tell you that chronic stress and elevated cortisol are wreaking havoc on the weight, memory, mood, and sex drive of millions of women. Our modern lifestyle has turned us into stress-cases who would rather go on Facebook than have sex with our partners. The worst part is that cortisol has the power to throw the other main hormones—estrogen, testosterone, thyroid—out of whack.

2. Yoga Conquers Cravings

You might be surprised to learn that the way to banish food cravings is not with meager 100-calorie snacks or the latest "Lose weight!" bar. In fact, it's managing your stress and cortisol levels, and the downstream benefit is fewer cravings for the carb-of-the-day.

Lower your cortisol, manage your stress, lower your glucose levels, and you'll see your cravings disappear. Massage and acupuncture have both been shown to lower stress, and so have low-impact exercises such as yoga. Although stress may keep you up at night now, getting at least seven hours of shut-eye per night will also help you regulate cortisol levels and stay on the right cortisol schedule—a burst in the morning to wake you up, and then a slow taper off over the course of the day that aids relaxation.

3. Yoga Is Superb Exercise

Unlike high-impact running, which increases cortisol, yoga lowers it. I've been a runner my entire life, but after adding to yoga to my routine, I lost weight, gained energy, and actually felt rejuvenated instead of depleted after my workouts. For stressed-out people, yoga provides a form of exercise that prevents hormones from going haywire and keeps cortisol in check.

4. Yoga Makes Your Breath Beautiful

The focus on breath and the meditative aspect of yoga also help change the way your mind interprets stress, leading to lowered cortisol levels and a calmer day-to-day. Yoga can be a serious workout, yes, but it can also be a quiet moment to yourself. *Ahh-omm.*

5. Yoga Upgrades Awareness

It's my opinion that body awareness is at an all-time low. Women are more likely to indulge a sugar craving than they are to set an earlier bedtime because they have never had a chance to get to know their own personal needs and rhythms. Becoming intimately familiar with your body's flexibility, breath, and the quietness (or lack thereof) of mind is a sorely under-recognized benefit of yoga.

One of the most important types of awareness that yoga emphasizes is that of your breath. *Pranayama* is the breathing technique of yoga that is said to increase physical and psychological performance. Deep breathing on its own has been proven to reduce stress and improve heart rate variability, but when you combine it with deep stretching, balance, and muscle-building? That's one heck of a recipe.

6. Yoga Amplifies the Happy Brain Chemicals

Have you ever talked to someone who practices yoga? I bet you've heard them say something to the effect of "I just feel so good after I do yoga." They're not just talking about the pride that comes from completing 90 minutes of Bikram. Yoga has been shown to raise your serotonin, the happy brain chemical responsible for mood, sleep, and appetite. Women have 52 percent less serotonin than men, according to my friend Daniel Amen, so that may be just one of the reasons we see fewer dudes on the mat—women need yoga to balance our serotonin, feel buoyant, sleep soundly, and put down the fork.

When you increase body awareness, one of the greatest benefits is the knowledge of how your actions affect your health. Rather than overeating, you remember how bad you felt last time you binged on ice cream. Yoga also teaches us how to recognize and forgive ourselves for bad habits. Instead of the depressing cycle of eat-guilt-eat, we learn to let our past transgressions go, and pave the way for better, healthier life choices.

7. Yoga Freshens Up Your Blood and Organs

The twisting, bending, and micro-adjustments of yoga keep your spine and joints strong and supple. Can you touch your toes? Getting to know your flexibility and physical limits can provide some enlightening insight into your own physical health. B. K. S. Iyengar tells us that yoga squeezes your organs like a sponge, removing the stale blood so that fresh, oxygenated blood can rush in when you release your twist. Maintaining your energy, flexibility, and strength using movements like these keeps exercise an option long into old age.

8. Yoga Is Good Medicine

Ayurveda is an ancient medical system of India that is based on the use of food, botanicals, meditation, and movement such as yoga. The Sanskrit term literally translates to "scripture for longevity." To me, Ayurveda is the *true* fountain of youth.

It promotes a lifestyle that is designed for not just a long life, but a happy life. Although starting a yoga practice doesn't mean you have to wear flowing clothes and grow dreadlocks, it does often result in new ways of thinking about yourself, your environment, and the relationship between the two.

9. Yoga Is Self-Love

There are certain habits and practices woven into the yogi's lifestyle that promote longevity and happiness, such as eating whole, seasonal foods, wearing comfortable clothes that are made out of natural fibers, and supplementing your lifestyle with botanicals that make you feel better, lighter, and happier. When you start doing things for yourself that create such positive effects—from weight loss to a sunnier mood—it's addicting, in the best sense of the word. If I could, I would prescribe "self-love" of this nature to every single person I meet.

You were born with intrinsic knowledge of how to heal. Somehow, cultural distortions and conditioning derailed you. Radical self-acceptance and self-love are your birthright, and you can reclaim them.

Healthy and Hormonally Balanced: Your Wabi-Sabi Approach

I struggled for many years to heal my own hormonal problems naturally by using the best science, and then I brought my carefully crafted protocols to the women I served. As a gynecologist, teacher, wife, mom, scientist, and yoga teacher, I spent years formulating, synthesizing, and testing a comprehensive plan for hormonal problems. It's my life's mission—to bring the fruits of my study, inquiry, and obsession with neuro-endocrine optimization to help other women feel balanced again.

Just as hormonal imbalance can be a vicious cycle that directly affects body image, hormonal balance can be the exact, wonderful opposite. Yoga is an important ingredient for me, as well as for hundreds of my patients, in our search for perfect health. It fits my exacting requirements for a recommended treatment: it's natural, proven, and effective. Yoga lowers cortisol, reduces inflammation, improves flexibility and circulation, raises awareness, and, when followed properly, increases forgiveness. All of these translate into a more positive body image and a healthier vessel for that hard-working brain.

Over time with yoga, we hone the ability to simply watch our actions and reactions without getting too involved. We develop a kind of spiritual toolkit that prepares us for dealing with our own particular body image baggage. Instead of spending hours obsessing about arm fat, you simply notice this as a thought and don't get involved. Instead of hating yourself for eating five after-dinner cookies, you forgive yourself. Overexercising becomes unnecessary simply because you are so attuned to your body that it doesn't feel good. Yoga provides specific tools that ground us in more meaningful self-inquiry than the number on the bathroom scale. It's one path off the roller coaster of obsession with female fatness. Armed with these skills, self-loathing, obsession with fatness, and displaced aggression have the potential to melt away. Yoga allows us to right-size the cultural conditioning that tells us what we should look like. We know better, and not because we saw it on an infomercial. This knowledge comes from inside. It's not a miracle cure. But it's one that works.

Today, I use yoga to live longer, love better, laugh louder, keep my mind clear, and prevent the most common health concerns that I know we all face. Yoga provides me the balance of work and play, of mindfulness and escape, and of relaxation and challenge. It also helps me maintain a positive body image and wabi-sabi perspective, because I know I look and feel healthier when I stick to a regular yoga practice, and also because staying in touch with my body in such a complete way keeps me on the path to balance and joy.

References

J. Banasik, H. Williams, M. Haberman, S. E. Blank, and R. Bendel. "Effect of Iyengar Yoga Practice on Fatigue and Diurnal Salivary Cortisol Concentration in Breast Cancer Survivors." *Journal of the American Academy of Nurse Practitioners* 23, 3 (2011): 135–142.

R. L. Bijlani, R. P. Vempati, R. K. Yadav, R. B. Ray, V. Gupta, R. Sharma, N. Mehta, and S. C. Mahapatra. "A Brief but Comprehensive Lifestyle Education Program Based on Yoga Reduces Risk Factors or Cardiovascular Disease and Diabetes Mellitus." *Journal of Alternative and Complementary Medicine* 11, 2 (2005): 267–274.

E. S. Epel, E. H. Blackburn, J. Lin, et al. "Accelerated Telomere Shortening in Response to Life Stress." *Proceedings of the National Academy of Sciences, USA* 101, 49 (2004): 17312–17315.

A. Gopal, S. Mondal, A. Gandhi, S. Arora, and J. Bhattacharjee. "Effect of integrated yoga practices on immune responses in examination stress—A preliminary study." *International Journal of Yoga* 4, 1 (2011): 26–32.

D. S. Khalsa, D. Amen, C. Hanks, N. Money, and A. Newberg. "Cerebral Blood Flow Changes During Chanting Meditation." *Nuclear Medicine Communications* 30, 12, (2009): 956–961.

B. G. Kalyani, G. Venkatasubramanian, R. Arasappa, N. P. Rao, S. V. Kalmady, R. V. Behere, H. Rao, M. K. Vasudey, and B. N. Gangadhar. "Neurohemodynamic Correlates of 'OM' Chanting: A Pilot Functional Magnetic Resonance Imaging Study." *International Journal of Yoga* 4, 1 (2011): 3–6.

R. Nidhi, V. Padmalatha, R. Nagarathna, and A. Ram. "Effect of a Yoga Program on Glucose Metabolism and Blood Lipid Levels in Adolescent Girls with Polycystic Ovary Syndrome." *International Journal of Gynaecology and Obstetrics* 118, 1 (2012): 37–41.

J. A. Smith, T. Greer, T. Sheets, and S. Watson. "Is There More to Yoga Than Exercise?" *Alternative Therapies in Health and Medicine* 17, 3 (2011): 22–29.

K. Upadhyay Dhungel, V. Malhotra, D. Sarkar, and R. Prajapati. "Effect of Alternate Nostril Breathing Exercise on Cardiorespiratory Functions." *Nepal Medical College Journal* 10, 1 (2008): 25–27.

S. Telles, P. Raghuraj, S. Maharana, and H. R. Nagendra. "Immediate Effect of Three Yoga Breathing Techniques on Performance on a Letter-Cancellation Task." *Perceptual and Motor Skills* 04, 3 Pt 2 (2007): 1289–1296.

J. West, C. Otte, K. Geher, J. Johnson, and D. C. Mohr. "Effects of Hatha Yoga and African Dance on Perceived Stress, Affect, and Salivary Cortisol." *Annals of Behavioral Medicine* 28, 2 (2004): 114–118.

··

Sara Gottfried, MD, is a natural hormone expert, Harvard-educated physician, keynote speaker, and author of *New York Times* bestseller *The Hormone Cure: Reclaim Balance, Sleep, Sex Drive and Vitality Naturally with the Gottfried Protocol* (Simon & Schuster, 2013). For the past twenty years, Dr. Gottfried has been dedicated to helping women and men feel at home in their bodies with natural hormone balancing through her virtual medicine practice and online learning center, the Gottfried Institute. www.SaraGottfriedMD.com

HOW SHAME FOUND ME ON THE YOGA MAT

Marianne Elliott

What do my tight hips say about me? That I'm sexually repressed? That my second chakra is blocked? That I don't know how to let go? That I'm not fit to be a yoga teacher? That I'm flawed in some fundamental way? That I'm not worthy of love and belonging?

That's what shame would have me believe.

As a yoga teacher, I sometimes fall into the trap of believing my body ought to be perfect. How are people supposed to believe in the benefits of yoga if I've been practicing all these years and yet I still catch a common cold every winter or struggle to get out of bed some mornings because my back hurts?

My sensible, rational mind tells me that it's in my humanity that I'm most useful as a teacher, that I have more to offer the real people who show up to my yoga courses because I too wake up with aches or sniffles some days. And my heart knows this. But the need to be perfect is persistent, and wherever there is perfectionism, for me there also is shame—and body shame runs deep.

Perfectionism

A couple of years ago I went to a yoga workshop led by a visiting international teacher. He's well-known and highly respected, and several of my yogi friends had recommended him. He sounded like the kind of teacher I could learn a lot from, so although he taught in a style that I don't practice regularly, I went along.

The first morning, after dragging myself out of the house at 5:30 AM, I found myself on my mat in a setting that, although in some ways familiar, was in many other ways quite foreign to me. To start with, the teacher was a man, which I wasn't used to. He yelled instructions across the room.

"Straighten that leg!" he called to the person behind me. "Straighten that leg!"

I glanced back to see that the person behind me was in a pose in which, according to my experience and training, forcing the leg to straighten before the hamstring is ready could harm the lower back.

My mind was suddenly busy as I assessed whether or not—in my opinion—each of the cues the teacher yelled out across the room was safe for the student at which it was directed. I wasn't doing this because I wanted to be right, but because I wanted to know whether I could trust the teacher—whether I could give myself into his care and follow his directions.

The shouted instructions were making it hard for me to stay connected to my inner teacher. But eventually I was able to let go of my need to take care of everyone else in the room and relax into my own breath and body. Things were going well until he decided to direct his attention at me.

He approached my mat as I gently eased my body into a complex twisting forward bend, one that demanded a little more openness in the hips than was available to me at six in the morning.

"Why is your knee there?" he asked. "Why don't you lower the knee?"

"It doesn't seem to want to lower this morning," I replied, not yet too disconcerted. I'd been in many classes when my knee wasn't ready to lower, and teachers had generally left it at that.

Not this teacher. He sat down beside me and shook my knee with his hand.

"Tight," he declared. "You are very tight."

In case there is any ambiguity, he wasn't saying tight as though it was a compliment or even a neutral observation. It was clear from his tone and expression that tight was *not* what my hip was supposed to be. He slapped at my knee a few times in what appeared to be an attempt to convince my hip to suddenly release and the knee to lower.

The slapping didn't produce the results he was hoping for. Instead, I felt a surge of heat to my face. My heart began to beat faster, and I suddenly realized I was about to burst into tears. I started breathing even more deeply and closed my eyes in an effort to stave off the tears. Maybe my closed eyes and deep breathing looked like a profound yogic moment to him, though, because he said, "Yes, yes. Very good. Keep breathing and this tightness will go away." Much to my relief, he then went away. The tightness, however, remained.

Then the tears came, and despite the many tears I've shed on my yoga mat, these surprised me. Tears sometimes come as I breathe my way into a deeper opening in a pose and, as I do, let go of emotions I've been holding and carrying in my body. I've cried tears of frustration on my mat, when I keep banging into myself no matter which path I try to take around. I've even cried tears of joy—when my body and breath come together to take me to a new place of freedom, clarity, beauty, and love on my mat. Grief, fear, frustration, relief, joy, even anger —I've come to recognize and eventually welcome all those tears.

But these were tears of shame.

Shame: The Shadow of Perfection

The work of Dr. Brené Brown has helped me recognize shame. Shame, says Dr. Brown, is "the intensely painful feeling that we are unworthy of love and belonging." [1] It's the most primitive human emotion we all feel and, she says, if left to its own devices, shame can destroy lives. It leads us to try to hide the parts of us that we fear may render us unlovable and tells us that we are the only ones who feel this way.

Once I knew how to recognize it, I saw that shame was hiding everywhere. And because so much shame is attached to our bodies, shame inevitably shows up on the yoga mat.

Like so many people, I have been raised in a culture that is rife with messages of shame about my body. From as soon as we are old enough to look out the window of the car or watch television, we are bombarded with images of how our bodies are supposed to look and—the corollary—how wrong our bodies are. Too fat, too skinny, too brown, too white, too scarred, too real. At a certain point in my teens, my body was simultaneously too skinny (for breasts) and too fat (for ballet).

Yoga: A Path to Uncover Our Worthiness

Then I began to practice yoga. I came to yoga because I was desperate. I returned from two years doing human rights monitoring in the Gaza Strip, my body weighed down with the grief and anger I had gathered up there and, not knowing what else to do with it, carried home to New Zealand. Within weeks of my return, my little sister was blindsided by grief and rushed home to New Zealand too. So there we both were, uprooted and adrift; we found a house by the sea and moved in together. We were unsure of how to breathe, what to trust, and how to find our way back into the sunlight, onto dry land.

Eventually, I found a yoga class, in a dusty community hall on the beach. I found a gentle-spoken teacher who pulled blankets, bolsters, blocks, and straps from a storage cupboard every Wednesday night and made tea for us after class. I found simple poses held long enough to feel my body and my breath, and slow, deep, restorative poses in which to cry softly.

In the decade that followed, I continued to explore yoga, learning to be patient and compassionate with my own body and, little by little, I began to appreciate my body for what it could do. It could hold me in a balancing pose and carry me through a flowing sequence of standing poses. My arms grew stronger and that mattered more than whether or not they looked good in an evening gown, especially since I never wore evening gowns. My legs grew strong and that mattered more than whether or not there was cellulite on my thighs.

And even more profoundly, yoga **gave** me a tool with which to turn toward my own shadows and to embrace what I met there with love— even when it was not what I thought I "should" find. Yoga gave me a practice to see my own worthiness and embrace my whole self. As I shone the light of yoga into the places I had long hidden in my body and my being, I loosened the grip of shame.

Layers of Shame

But shame can be insidious, and as I began to shed some of my shameful feelings about my body, I accumulated new ones. Despite my excellent teachers, whose wisdom was always swimming against the stream of everything I had learned before I arrived in their class, I picked up a whole new set of ideas about what my body should be able to do. Those damn hips that simply wouldn't release into the deceptively named "Easy Cross-legged pose" became a source of shame for me. This was especially true when teachers suggested that tight hips were a sign of an emotional unwillingness or inability to let go.

Oh, how I tried to let go.

Maybe what my "tight" hips say about me is that I like to run long distances, up to fifty kilometers in a week, and that I walk from my house to work every day and then back up the long hill again in the evening. Maybe they say that I'm a writer as well as a yoga teacher, and spend more time at my desk than on my yoga mat. Maybe my "tight" hips say something about the angle of my femoral anteversion, the orientation of my acetabulum, the shape of my femoral neck, or the elasticity my iliofemoral ligament. Maybe there's nothing wrong with any of those things.

Maybe the "tension" I'm holding in my hips is not a sign of a deep-seated emotional, spiritual, and psychological failure.

Today I find that possibility easy to entertain, but when I encountered Mr. "You-are-very-tight," I was still in the grip of body perfectionism and its shadow—body shame.

Almost certainly, the teacher who tapped at my knee and told me part of me was very tight had no idea that in my mind having tight hips was closely correlated to failing to be emotionally or spiritually evolved. Each of us carries our own secret pockets of body shame, some of them harder to spot than others. So how much responsibility can a yoga teacher take for creating a shame-free yoga space?

Is Shame Different?

A male yoga teacher friend of mine, in response to my story of hip-shame and tears on the mat, proposed that there was a difference between a teacher judging us and "making us feel shame," on the one hand, and "triggering old shame" on the other by testing us in uncomfortable situations.

If it's okay, even good, for yoga classes (and by extension yoga teachers) to trigger the release of other emotions, then why is triggering the release (or habitual response) of old shame any different?

Yoga is the path through, rather than around, our shadows. So I can see my friend's point. If this teacher's style, tone, words, or action reconnected me to old body shame, then he helped create a powerful learning opportunity for me. There is no doubt that through this experience I became more aware of a pattern of shame I've embodied.

As I told this friend, *it seemed despite seeking out compassionate yoga teachers, I still carry the hard taskmaster, the shrill critic, within me. I don't think this teacher shamed me. He just triggered my own internal critic, who does a very good job of making me feel not good enough or not worthy, which is pretty much my definition of shame. That internal critic gets a lot less airtime these days than in the past, so it caught me off guard—very much off guard! But it was a useful learning experience.*

So, if I was carrying these old feelings of shame with me, and if they needed to be released or at least recognized, then didn't the teacher do what all yoga teachers aspire to do—create an opportunity for me to learn and grow and deepen in my yoga and my life?

In one sense he did. But shame is a very powerful emotion. It has the capacity to paralyze us, and it certainly has the potential to send an otherwise curious new yoga student away from a class with no intention of ever returning.

Shame-Free Yoga: Is It Possible?

It is for this reason that I am especially mindful, as a yoga teacher and as a human, of the most common shame triggers. Sadly, the body is one of the most common sites of shame.

I agree with my friend: when (and only when) a teacher comes to know a student well, and once that student knows and trusts the teacher, there is a powerful space in which a teacher may gently encourage and support a student to extend themselves beyond their comfort zone. A wise and intuitive teacher can have a good sense of what each student is capable of doing, which may be more than that student suspects.

I've certainly had yoga teachers encourage me to try poses or go to places in my practice that I believed to be beyond me. When I trust those teachers enough, I'll go even where I believe I cannot go.

In my case, it may be that the teacher had such strong intuition that he saw that I not only carried "shame" baggage but that I had the strength, self-awareness, and support to be able to process that shame. He may even have knowingly poked my weak spot to show me what was lying beneath the surface. If he did, he certainly created a profound learning opportunity for me.

But it takes careful judgment to know when a student has the support and tools to process a stored emotion as strong as shame without creating new shame. This is especially true because we generally don't know what is going on in someone's life outside the yoga class, nor do we know what experiences they may have had that will profoundly affect how they receive and interpret our words and actions.

The bottom line for me is that before we can skillfully engage with external teachers, we need to recover our core relationship with our inner teacher, the part of us that knows what is best for our own body. This relationship is healed through love and trust, so my primary goal as a yoga teacher is to create an environment in which people can meet their own bodies with love and learn to trust their own body wisdom.

I do what I can to avoid feeding or triggering body shame in my classes by—among other things—choosing language that welcomes and honors every body in the room, avoiding language that privileges one kind of body or one experience of a pose over any others, by reminding students that they know best what is right for them and their body, and by asking for permission before I touch people.

But I also accept that at the end of the day I cannot control what arises in people as they practice with me. I'm sure there are people who have been in my classes who could tell a story about how my choice of words or adjustment triggered their own feelings of shame.

Shame is such a widely shared experience and can leave such deep wounds that all yoga teachers and yoga students are likely to face it at some point. I only hope that I can create a safe and supportive environment in which my students can experience whatever may arise as they practice yoga.

As a yoga teacher, my commitment is to be mindful of that context when I teach. My commitment is to ask permission before I touch a student and then when I do touch someone, to do so in a way that gives them the opportunity to control the encounter as much as possible.

My commitment is to invite people to take control of their own practice and to feel free to choose how to move or not move their bodies. My commitment is to be mindful of my language and of the assumptions I might make about people based on how their bodies look.

My commitment is to remember that every person who walks into a yoga class or uses one of my yoga videos has their own long history of being told that their body needs to change, to be different. My commitment is to remember the power I have as a yoga teacher and to use that power in a way that honors the first *yama*, *ahimsa*—to do no harm.

My commitment is to teach in a way that, as far as possible, reinforces positive experiences of and messages about our bodies. My commitment is to teach without shame.

1. Brené Brown. "Shame v. Guilt." www.brenebrown.com/2013/01/14/2013114shame-v-guilt-html/ (accessed March 2014).

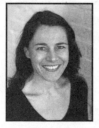 **Marianne Elliott** is a writer, human rights advocate, and yoga teacher. She's the author of *Zen Under Fire* (Sourcebooks) about her work with the UN in Afghanistan, and how she found peace (and yoga) even in the midst of war. Her 30 Days of Yoga online courses help people take care of themselves so they can do their good work in the world. She is a senior leader for Off the Mat, Into the World. www.marianne-elliott.com

Author photo by Luca Putnam.

TOO MUCH IS NOT ENOUGH

Dr. Melody Moore

I grew up in a family, and in a culture, where I came to perceive that what mattered about me and what was lovable about me was the way that I looked. I believed that if I were thin and pretty, I would be loved. And that if I was fat, I was in sin. Yes, sin. I was taught that gluttony was an abomination to God and filled in the blanks from there. Granted, I came to these conclusions based on misperceptions and illusions about what was important to my dad about my mom and to my family about me. Of course I was wrong, but the idea that my worth was measured by my weight was deeply ingrained in my psyche. It would have taken a miracle for me to believe that who I am and the way that I treat myself, and therefore others, are what matter. I was certain that if I didn't look beautiful, I would not be loved. And that if I was not loved, I would not survive. Ironically, I almost missed out on my life because I was so concerned with my appearance.

This struggle to accept my body was assuredly going to be never-ending. I would never achieve the perfect physical form, and as long as I was convinced that I would not be loved until I was perfect, I would continue to be plagued by a limiting belief about myself. I was too much—too fat, too big, too unworthy.

My own body hatred subsided after I moved away from home to college, which allowed me an opportunity to release myself from my self-induced competition with my mom and sister to out-thin them. My older sister had a fierce battle with anorexia beginning in 1997. She was never clinically treated, and for years her symptoms overwhelmed me with feelings of helplessness, anger, and fear. I have always been the opposite of her, so in many ways her diagnosis allowed me to find more acceptance of my body, not less. It also set me up for a path toward convincing others that they are worthy of a full life of purpose, meaning, and connection. Starting with my own.

Pura Vida

In 2001, my mom chose a yoga retreat called Pura Vida, in Costa Rica, for our family's annual vacation. None of us had ever stepped foot onto a yoga mat. Who gets to have her first yoga class in the mountains of Costa Rica? This girl. I was fascinated by yoga and a little bit afraid of it. My teacher seemed so patient, whole-hearted, and full of joy. After a weeklong immersion and introduction to the practice, I invited the teacher, Srutih, to call me if she ever came to Dallas. A few weeks later, she called to ask if she could move in with me for three months to help some friends open a studio.

So my introduction to the practice was really through having an in-home yoga teacher. Sharing my home with Srutih meant that I was able to delve into yoga, chanting, and meditation right in my own living room. At the time, I had no idea what a privileged position I was in. When Srutih moved out, I continued my daily yoga practice at Sunstone, the studio she helped to open. I went every day, without much inner negotiation. Clearly, I was still abiding by the idea that workouts must be done every day, no matter what. I had integrated this nonnegotiable attitude from my mom, who prioritized her exercise above, well, everything.

Her mindset was that she would be easier to tolerate after she allowed her body to release pent-up stress and aggression. My interpretation of what felt like a compulsion to exercise was that she valued thinness and prettiness above all else. And, because I was her daughter,

I thought she not only valued her own thinness, but mine too. In fact, I fell completely into the delusion that what was lovable and worthy about me was being pretty, which in my mind meant being thin. I was wrong. The miracle of yoga was its capacity to turn not only my body but my thoughts right side up.

It took some time, though. For the first five years of practicing, I only knew yoga to be a workout, and a very good one at that. I loved sweating it out, I loved the feeling of *savasana* after a long physical detox, and I loved that my body was looking leaner and more toned. I was completely unaware that I was becoming more present to my breath, less reactive, more patient, and more open to experiencing my emotions.

Practice Makes Practice

Yoga eventually had its way with me. It took navigating through a series of styles, studios, and teachers, and staying committed to a daily practice for several years for me to connect to the fact that what had become my way of life had also become my way of living. I realized, around year seven of practice, that yoga was the instrument through which I was finding emotional freedom, spiritual clarity, and certainly body acceptance. It was a gradual process, and a subtle one too. There were moments of poignancy after about a five-year gestation process of what I now can refer to as striving for perfection in the pose. One came to me during a class by a teacher named Lisa Coyle, who dropped this little pearl during a Sun Salutation B vinyasa: "Every exhale is an opportunity to forgive." While I have no doubt that I had heard many iterations of this concept during what were, by that time, hundreds of hours on the mat, that day something clicked. Yoga then became a spiritual practice. It became a way of living that allowed me to be present.

Through this attentiveness to the rate and pace of my inhales and exhales, I learned to be so present to the moment that I had no choice but to let go of what had been or could become. On my mat, it was impossible to time travel back to the past or forward into the future, when I was so alive and attuned to that very particular, once-in-a-lifetime inhale or exhale of breath. And just like that, I started paying attention to what else yoga was offering me, what other nectar I had drawn from the practice. I became invested in learning how what I had cultivated on the mat could be carried over into my life off the mat.

I realized that the time I had dedicated to being on the mat had allowed me to release years of tension, conscious and unconscious, physical and emotional. My yoga practice offered me tools to ground, center, and find balance. More than anything, my practice allowed me to recognize the connections that I have to everyone around me and to the universe. My practice became the place where I felt closest to God. Not the understanding of God that I had formerly been introduced to as one who punishes gluttony, among other sins, but God the source of love and the wisdom that creates and connects and conspires in each of our favors. As my practice became spiritual, I became a seeker. Not only did I seek to feel more into the subtleties of *asana*, but I began to pursue the purpose of my life as well. I integrated the capacity to rely on my own breath to determine when to modify and whether to intensify, both on and off the yoga mat. A decade into daily practice, there came to be a fluidity in what was "on" and what was "off" the mat. As I recognized the delight in letting go of perfecting a pose in order to find the feeling inside of it, I came to live in alignment with that realization. And then it happened: a realization that I am holy, connected, supported, and worthy. Not at year one, or five, but a decade later. Because practice makes practice.

Behold the Body Temple

In my seeking, I found that yoga had made me feel whole. I found that through the connection of my mind to my body through the breath, I had actually been repairing the severed cords between my heart, head, and gut. Through seeking to find alignment in each physical pose, I had also been learning how to find alignment in what I was feeling, doing, thinking, and saying. Yoga had brought me into my integrity. I was not in parts, I was not in conflict, I was not creating tension for myself, my psyche, or my body. In fact, I was in balance. At least, I was able to use my core resources to come back into balance, again and again, after coming too close to the edges and too uncomfortable with misalignment. Not only was I in balance with myself, I strove to be in balance with the flow of the universe, with the grace of God. As I found courage, I learned to surrender to this grace.

It was actually a side effect, not a conscious objective, that I was not viewing my body negatively or putting much emphasis, if any, on my external appearance. Because I was not seeing my appearance as needing to shift or change, be thinner or more beautiful, the natural progression of self-love was that I let go of the illusion that my worth was measured by my size. I did not purposefully set out or even consciously determine to create a positive body image through yoga; it just arrived as a byproduct of all of the other gifts that the practice bestowed. *As my yoga practice became a prayer, my body became a temple.* I began to honor it as the keeper of my sweet soul, and as the guardian of what had become a recognition and a celebration of the light within me.

I realized that I felt good about my body after going to Hawaii with my bestie, Chris, who turned to me on our last day and said, "You know, it has been really lovely and so easy to be around someone who doesn't say anything negative about their body. I don't think I have ever been around a woman, especially in a swim suit, who is not pejorative about her weight or size, or about other women's bodies." He recognized what I knew. I had completely let go of picking apart my appearance. I used the mirrors at some yoga studios to reset alignment from time to time, but other than that, I didn't ever stand in front of a mirror and, part by part, examine what needed to shrink, expand, or change. He was right—what he witnessed was my truth.

Through yoga, I found that I really liked who I had become, and in so doing, I had stopped emphasizing how I looked. I recognized, through my practice, that my emotions served as the best compass for my happiness. My yoga practice literally had transformed the lens through which I saw myself, my capacity, my lovability, and my worth. Through yoga, I was able to feel whatever emotion was arising in my body without immediately wanting out of it. I was able to tolerate feelings and even to welcome them. For probably the first time in my life, I was able to be with whatever feeling came, without fear that it would kill me. And so I learned to trust myself. I needed this trust in order to feel safe. I needed to feel safe in order to feel like I would survive. I needed to survive in order to trust that I could thrive.

Yoga is a *practice*, it is not a *perfect*, and there is no perfecting it. However, in the letting go of that attempt, for me, there became what yoga teacher Tias Little has called "a striving for imperfection." In surrendering outcomes of poses, there opens up a possibility for feeling, blossoming, and awakening. I had so many years and layers and levels of defenses built up around me from childhood, it took me a decade to break them down to the point that I felt fully alive to the awareness that I could breathe. I did not need to be reactive; I could witness my own behavior. I could stop comparing myself to others and hold myself with so much kindness and compassion that there would be no space for shame about my body, my past behaviors, or anything else. Yoga brought me into a sense not only of being connected to myself but to everything around me as well. Most of all, yoga brought me back to God.

Giving It Away

"Let the beauty we love be what we do.
There are hundreds of ways to kneel and kiss the ground."—Rumi

I was so full of gratitude for the practice that I began to feel like I was out of balance by not giving it away. I was taking and taking and not giving, and I finally had to find a way to share with others how I had benefited from the practice of yoga. This was especially poignant because, as a psychologist who specializes in the treatment of girls and women with disordered eating and negative body image, I had done years of deep listening. I had been given extraordinary training and had a sincere wish to be helpful. But I knew that only offering psychotherapy to a client who has severed the cords between their mind and their body, often to the point of near death, was not enough to help them thrive.

If I could help them out of their heads, out of their thinking, and into their bodies, into their feeling, they would build a container for themselves that would allow them to trust what they feel. This trust would allow them to rely on their gut wisdom to honor their emotions and to respond to their hunger. Not all of those who struggle with eating disorders are striving for their idea of a perfect body, but everyone who struggles with disordered eating is acting out their emotions through their self-perception and / or their food behavior. Bringing yoga into treatment would allow a reconnection of mind and body, and body and breath, and through breath, gut and intuition, in a way that I knew would be healing.

My clients had overemphasized their appearance as being a measure of their worth to the point of, in many cases, the brink of death. In attempting to help them trust themselves enough to actually experience emotion, in the moment, as it arose, no matter what, I had to find a way to incorporate yoga, the physical practice of *asana*. Emotions are physical sensations stored as peptides in cells in the body. Those who struggle with disordered eating have become severed at the places where the mind and body connect. Those with anorexia do not eat when they are hungry; they starve because it is a way out of feeling. Those with binge eating disorder or bulimia do not overeat because they are hungry; they overeat because they are trying to soothe themselves through what they do not think they can tolerate feeling. Eating becomes a way of soothing, and body hatred and distortion become a way of defending against discomfort. Yoga is a tool by which we can develop the capacity to sit with and through discomfort, and eventually even "greet it at the door laughing" to paraphrase Rumi's poem, "The Guest House."

To bring clients more fully into their whole selves, to help them stop seeing themselves as individual pieces and separate parts to be perfected, I envisioned and created a collaboration of yoga, holistic nutrition, and psychotherapy called the Embody Love Center. At our holistic treatment center for those struggling with disordered eating and negative body image, clients experience integrated treatments that can bring them into what I believe is a possibility for self-acceptance and true self-love and respect. Through yoga, clients are able to feel the ground underneath them and know support. They are able to witness and experience themselves as capable and whole, as acceptable and worthy. They are able to tolerate what they feel, and they are able to integrate their breath with their movement. One client (who is now a yoga teacher) shared with me after an early experience with yoga that by feeling her breath in her belly, she could feel hunger for the first time in a long time. To us both, her ability to sense and to honor her body's hunger signal seemed to be a miracle. Yoga had yoked her body to her mind, and from there, she had a chance, finally, to survive and to thrive.

Yoga offers us the capacity to be, to accept, to allow, to make room, to grow, to feel, to love, to let go. For me, this practice of imperfection allows me to be fully in love with the moments that life offers and fully accepting of whatever way that I arrive to them. Yoga has allowed me to live inside a body temple and to offer the same experience to others. I cannot imagine a more holy, more sacred, or more beautiful practice of living.

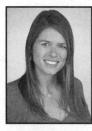 **Melody Moore, PhD,** is a clinical psychologist who specializes in recovery from eating disorders and negative body image through integrated treatment of psychotherapy, holistic nutrition, family therapy, and the healing practice of yoga. Dr. Moore founded the Embody Love Movement, a nonprofit whose vision is to create a world where all see and treat themselves, and therefore others, as lovable without condition. www.embodylovemovement.org

Author photo by Alayna MacPherson Photography.

MAYBE THE PROBLEM ISN'T MY BODY

Anna Guest-Jelley

When I was a little girl, my parents tried to get me to stick with a sport. Or get a sport to stick with me. Basically, they would take whatever worked.

But nothing did.

On my first day of softball practice, someone hit an errant ball, and it slammed into my back—hard. The fact that my back could somehow be toward the ball in this scenario is both beside the point and the entire point. All I remember is having the breath knocked out of me and the huge bruise I got. That was my last day of softball.

I didn't have the hand-eye coordination for tennis. And while I enjoyed swimming, I didn't have a competitive enough spirit to care about competing. So that's when my mom and I started aerobics. Oh, and it's also when I started Weight Watchers.

I was 12 years old.

Middle-Aged Ladies and Me

Being the only kid at both the Firm Factor (because, of course, what else could an aerobics place be called in the early nineties) and Weight

Watchers was a heady mix of pride (look how I can bust this move, la-dies!) and shame (OMG, where are the other kids?).

The day I saw my middle-school math teacher at Weight Watch-ers pretty much sums up the entire experience. I was horrified that she'd seen me stripped down to my spandex (because, of course, you wouldn't want the pesky weight of jeans negatively affecting the 0.2 pounds you'd lost that week). As the only girl in a sea of middle-aged women, I wasn't particularly hard to spot. I remember seeing her first, and trying to hide behind my mom—subtly, of course. I mean, I was 12. I had my dignity to consider.

I did my weigh-in, and I'd gotten to a magical moment: 10 pounds lost. When you hit these milestones in Weight Watchers back in the day, they gave you something cool (probably even more so to a kid)— a sticker, a bookmark, something that looks like those awards you'd win on field day at school (which had never graced my palm before, of course).

Naturally, my mom wanted me to stay, even though I wanted to get the h-e-double-hockey-sticks out of there after seeing my teacher. I think Mom was hoping the pride of a literal gold star would moti-vate me to lose even more weight and stay skinny forever. Little did she know how unmotivated I am by things like that (or maybe she to-tally knew and was hoping that the support of the weight-loss-obsessed crowd would buoy me).

So, after oh-so-discreetly pleading with her to let me leave, I took my seat in the back. If you haven't been to one of these meetings, think church revival meets infomercial meets AA meeting (without the blessed anonymity). Women (almost always women) sit in rows not un-like pews, hear a sermon from their "leader," and then have the oppor-tunity to confess their sins ("I ate two candy bars this week!"), repent (committing to the weight loss theme of the week), and do an altar call (delighting in their food piety or pledging to reform—starting on Mon-day).

It was the altar call I was particularly dreading that week. As some-one who was owed an award for leaving her 10 pounds behind, I wanted my recognition. But I also rebuffed it and didn't want to call attention to myself (since I was still hoping beyond hope that my teacher hadn't seen me, though she would have had to have been struck blind to not see the only kid in the small, albeit jam-packed, room).

Also, I'll admit it: a part of me wanted her to know. I mean, I'd lost 10 pounds, dang it! What other 12-year-old was busting their ass as hard? I sure didn't see any others in the room, now, did I? And just think: If I could work this hard here, imagine what I could do in school. Right, teacher friend?

So I tentatively raised my hand when our leader asked people to share their successes of the week. And as I proclaimed my 10 pounds lost, I locked eyes with my teacher just at the moment I was handed my award, which if you didn't look at the writing on the front looked like I was carrying around a blue ribbon for first place in relay (with a gold star to boot!).

I can still see her face now, a mix of pity, sadness, shame, and, well, begrudging happiness for me. I mean, I had lost 10 pounds. Who wouldn't celebrate that?

The Dreaded Tally

While Weight Watchers didn't mark the beginning of my weight-loss journey (more like a desperate attempt to end it after the apocalyptic warnings from my pediatrician that I was on the wrong end of the weight percentiles for kids, which horrified my tiny mother), it is a particularly notable stop along the way. Notable because, after "failing" (those 10 pounds were one of my last award ribbons), I didn't blame Weight Watchers. Instead, I blamed three things: (1) me, (2) my body, and (3) the fact that I hadn't yet found the right diet.

I just knew there had to be one out there that would work like you see on TV or in magazines. Before/after. Sinner/saint. So I kept looking. For the next fifteen-plus years, I tried every diet out there. At one point not too long ago, I tallied it up, and I came up with a list of sixty-five different diets I'd been on. And some of those (such as Weight Watchers), I was on multiple times over the years.

That's when it hit me: maybe, just maybe, a sixty-sixth diet wouldn't work either. Maybe, just maybe, I had this all bass-ackwards in the first place.

Mostly, I doubted that little seed of an idea because that's just how insidious diet culture is. There's nothing else in the world that people would try and fail more than sixty-five times, and keep blaming themselves for. I mean, if my Internet goes down even once, I don't blame myself. I'm immediately up in arms about how terrible my Internet provider is, even though it works smoothly 99.99 percent of the time. But diets continuing to not "work"? For twenty years? And in all varieties?

Obviously, I'm the one who's not doing something right.

When the Pain Came

In the background of all this dieting, I had a number of health problems. In middle school, I had chronic, unexplained stomach pain. I got a diagnosis of irritable bowel syndrome (IBS), but that's basically just the doctor's way of saying "your stomach hurts, but we don't really know why." The stomach pain eventually faded away, quickly forgotten by bigger dramas including moving to a new state, and thus school, for the start of eighth grade.

That is, until the migraines came.

In my junior year of high school, I started getting migraines—really bad ones. The kind that limit your vision to the extent that you start to wonder if it will ever come back. The kind with pain that can't be explained in words but only moans. The kind with flashing lights, nausea, and an inability to get comfortable in any position. Most days, I didn't even bother trying to take a nap because lying there in the dark, unable to sleep, was more painful than staying awake in the light.

These migraines quickly picked up frequency to the point that I had them every single day. Even now just thinking about it, my heart breaks. The amount of pain I suffered that year was, and is, incredible.

My parents took me to every doctor, and I tried every possible medication, test, and treatment—no matter how far-fetched—available. This was before high schools began to strictly monitor what students carry in their backpacks, so mine always had a bottle of Vicodin, which I would discreetly pop between classes in order to keep going.

None of those pills or tests ever really worked. After about a year, though, I found a regimen that helped—I was getting migraines "only" one or two times a week, rather than every day. And while that was an improvement, it wasn't enough. I was disillusioned, cynical, and both convinced that I'd always be in pain and determined not to let that happen.

Finding Yoga

When I went to college, I took things into my own hands. I knew that I had to find something, anything that would help me. I didn't want to live my college years, finally on my own like I'd been yearning for, the same way I did my last couple years of high school. So I started researching, and I found biofeedback, which is a technique that can help people with chronic pain. The roots of biofeedback are in meditation, so I began looking more into that.

When I read books about meditation and began practicing it, I knew I was home. I became able to feel a migraine coming on, stop and visualize my pain (my go-to image was always a squished-up angry red ball), and dissolve it. It didn't always go away completely, but it was definitely dramatically lessened. No prescription drug had ever given me such relief—particularly without the inevitable side effects.

A complete convert to the power of meditation, my reading brought me in short order to yoga. Even though I had still never found a form of movement I'd actually enjoyed, I knew I wanted to give yoga a try.

First of all, it wasn't a team sport. Score one for yoga.

Second of all, I could do it by myself, in the relative privacy of my dorm room. Score two for yoga.

I somehow got my hands on a yoga mat and a Rodney Yee VHS tape, and I popped it in when my roommate was in class. As I moved through the poses, I felt something I hadn't felt in a really long time— good. And even though my body didn't look even a little bit like Rodney Yee's, I knew I'd found something completely transformative for me.

Making the Connection

All through college and into graduate school, I mostly continued to feel better. I did have longish stints of chronic migraines two more times, but they were never quite as bad as the first one. Yoga and meditation helped. And, eventually, acupuncture changed everything for the better—and for the long run (knock on wood).

In the midst of all that healing, I began to yearn for another healing too. I started questioning, after all those years, whether or not I'd ever find the "right" diet for me, where I'd finally magically lose all that weight that had surely been the only block between me and an always-perfect, pain-free life. Because that's what all thin people have, right? Right...

As I broke through the idea that I would always have to be in pain, I also began to break through the idea that I would always have to be on a diet. At first this looked a lot like finding new ways to diet—seemingly more healthy ways, such as intense cleanses. This was before everyone and their brother began juicing, so it was still pretty out there.

When that didn't work (I'd lose 10 pounds in a week, then gain back 9.95 the next week once I started eating again), I sought out a nutritionist. After watching her lay out plastic food on a plate to illustrate portion sizes, I realized I needed an approach that didn't totally infantilize me. Fortunately, I found a nutrition therapist in my town who specialized in intuitive eating. Her questions about how I know when I'm hungry and full blew my mind. I spent months noting my satiety on a scale from 1 to 10 every time I ate.

Most meals and days, this felt like a guess. Although this process was difficult for me, after having trained myself for nearly twenty years to disengage from my hunger and satiety cues and eat by the external guidelines of a diet, I know that the only way I was able to engage with it at all was because of yoga.

Through yoga, I learned that when a yoga teacher asks you to "feel what's going on in your back leg in Warrior I," that's not a metaphor like I'd originally thought. Yoga taught me that it was possible to feel what was going on in my body—something I'd never experienced before because I'd been living pretty much exclusively in my head. And once I got a glimmer of what it's like to live in connection with my body, it was only a matter of time until I could apply those skills in other areas of my life, such as sensing when a migraine was coming on or noticing when I was hungry or full.

Maybe the Problem Isn't My Body

As I continued to work with reconnecting with my body's own internal wisdom about what was right for me to eat, I began to play with the notion that maybe my ideas about my yoga practice could also be transformed. Although I loved practicing, I'd been secretly thinking all along that I'd finally *really* get it once I turned into one of the skinny bendies I usually saw on the mat beside me in class. But then one day, I had this thought: "Wait a minute … what if the problem isn't my body? What if the problem is just that my teachers don't know how to teach me or other people with bigger bodies?"

It was that simple—but deeply profound for me—question that eventually helped me work up the courage to become a yoga teacher (or, at least, to go to teacher training and hope I didn't spontaneously combust because of being the biggest person in the room, by a long shot).

Curvy Yoga

After my initial teacher training, I knew I wanted to teach other curvy-bodied people like me. Slowly and informally, my message grew. I started by teaching my friends, then writing a blog that only two people read on a good day. My initial hunch turned out to be true: I wasn't the only curvy person out there who wanted to practice yoga. Far from it, actually.

Every week, my inbox fills with messages from people who never thought yoga was available to them because their body is far from the bodies we see practicing yoga on TV and on magazine covers. It also fills with messages from people who have been shamed in yoga classes, both implicitly and explicitly, for "not being able to keep up," for "just being too big for yoga," and any other number of insults and falsehoods.

But, thankfully, my inbox also fills more and more these days with messages from passionate and thoughtful teachers who want to make their classes accessible for people of all shapes and sizes. These teachers want their classes to be a place where everyone feels safe, welcome, and able to participate in a body-positive, noncompetitive environment.

This is what feels like my life's work: connecting these students and teachers and continuing to open up the conversation around how yoga can support the many of us who can benefit from (re)connecting with our bodies—both on and off the mat.

How Yoga Supports Body Image

Many, if not most, of us have disconnected from our bodies for various reasons. People with bigger bodies are told nearly everywhere they turn—the media, friends, family, doctors, public policy—that the only relationship that is okay to have with their body is one that's about control and changing a body that is deemed not yet good enough.

All of those messages are about shaming people into change, and that's not a strategy that works. Shame drives people into isolation and keeps them from getting the support they need. In other words, it does the opposite of motivating. And it certainly doesn't give people the tools they need to determine what their unique body actually needs.

Yoga that shows people they are the experts on their own experience can help them reestablish a body/mind connection. While someone else might be able to help you open the door of empowerment, it's ultimately an inside job. No one else empowers you. You empower yourself. And as that inner empowerment unfolds, you step into your agency and can begin to take compassionate action on your own behalf.

Yoga in action. You in action.

Set Free

By slowly learning how to feel what was going on in my body from the inside out on my yoga mat, I began to translate that off my mat. And the more I did that, the more clearly I knew what was right for me—and what wasn't. After more than two decades, I let go of my pattern of disordered eating and chronic dieting. I left a job that wasn't right for me and became an entrepreneur, working with Curvy Yoga full-time. I let go of friendships that weren't right for me. I set boundaries around my time and what I am and am not willing to do with it. And I finally gave myself permission to care for and love myself in the body I have today.

All of this would have been so improbable, if not impossible, without yoga. It's what gave me the confidence and know-how to turn away from the myriad messages coming at me every day to be different and look different than I do. And to do so with as much grace as I can muster—feeling good in my skin, despite the odds.

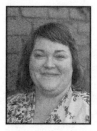

Anna Guest-Jelley is the founder and CEO (Curvy Executive Officer) of Curvy Yoga, a training and inspiration portal offering classes, workshops, teacher trainings, retreats, and lots of love and support to women of every size, age, and ability—in multiple countries and the majority of US states. Author of *Permission to Curve: Inspiring Poses for Curvy Yogis & Their Teachers*, Anna has been featured online and in print in the *Washington Post, US News & World Report, Southern Living, Vogue Italia, Yoga International, Yoga Journal*, and more. www.curvyyoga.com

Author photo by Vivienne McMaster.

PART TWO

On the Margins

Many of us can relate to feeling out of place or different at some point in our lives. This section explores feeling out of place or being "the other," whether it's being excluded from members of our peer culture, not falling within the narrow confines of the mainstream beauty ideal, or the expectation of the "yoga body." In fact, often that "outsider" status can refer to finding oneself on the margin of yoga culture itself.

The contributors in this section examine their experiences of standing on the margins, the roots of their outsider status, and how, with the cultivation of a consistent yoga practice, they were each able to come home to themselves. While the roots of their feelings of marginalization and isolation are varied, what they share in common is the key role the practice of yoga played and continues to play in bringing them into a space of wholeness.

Vytas Baskauskas shares the intimate and painful details of his heroin addiction, homelessness, and eventual imprisonment. Seeking solace, comfort, and connection through food, sex, and drugs was never enough. He shares how his yoga and meditation practice have helped fill his internal well and how the process of developing self-love is a daily practice, a work in progress.

Dianne Bondy's story is a tale of bravery and triumph. She candidly and openly shares her feelings of marginalization as related to her race and size. Because she had no role models to emulate or images to relate to, her sense of insecurity and isolation grew. Yoga provided the path to her self-awareness and acceptance. Ultimately, it allowed her to create a career to share these gifts by teaching yoga and challenging yoga stereotypes.

Carrie Barrepski's essay is a remarkable story of an inspiring and determined woman who has overcome obstacle after obstacle, never allowing her physical disabilities to define her. By modifying poses and listening to her body, she embarked on a yoga practice that allowed her to let go of shame and fear, as well as negative self-talk, and fully blossom in love and self-acceptance.

Practicing yoga was highly unlikely for Teo Drake, and it certainly wasn't love at first sight. His is a moving tale of coming to peace with a body that he had waged war on for most of his life, as well as a culture that told him his body was wrong. Over time, yoga became a pathway to compassion, sensitivity, and acceptance.

As a "short, middle-aged, average-looking Asian woman," Joni Yung doesn't look like a yoga cover model or the countless yoga stereotypes that exist about what a yoga practitioner looks like. And while this has challenged her body image, it hasn't stopped her from practicing or sharing her passion for yoga. Hers is a story about the changing face of yoga, mainstream yoga culture, and finding her voice amidst an identity crisis.

WORK IN PROGRESS

Vytas Baskauskas

"Twenty minutes," he tells me in a thick Oaxacan accent. I hang up the phone, grab my things, and hop in the car, hoping that this time his estimate is accurate but knowing deep down that it's going to be at least an hour before I feel relief.

Being dopesick is the worst feeling I've ever had to endure, and today is no different. My nose is running, my stomach is churning, my legs are flinching, and the urge to vomit is very close to being overpowering. It is this awful sickness that propels me into the ghetto of Los Angeles to meet my dealer. At this point, I've been strung out on heroin for the last two years and my addiction has progressed to a point where I don't do much else. Pretty much everything in my life is geared toward drugs: the getting, the using, the ways and means to get more.

As I wait anxiously for him to arrive, I feel the eyes on me. With each minute of waiting, the sickness gets worse. I can barely hold my bowels. My shirt is soaked with sweat. It's been forty minutes and I'm starting to worry that something happened. If he doesn't show, I'm fucked. Finally, after more than an hour, he picks me up and we go for a ride. I rarely have the exact amount of money, but today he takes pity and doesn't give me a hard time when I drop $17 on him for a $20 balloon. He spits the dope into my hand and drops me back off. I'm really struggling now. I gag a few times trying not to vomit. I can't run because I'll shit myself.

Hobbling to my car, I realize that I'd better fix here because I'm not going to make it home. A good junkie never goes anywhere without his supplies. I take out the spoon, cotton, and syringe. After a little cook, the needle is full of sweet brown liquid and I'm ready to feel relief. When I first started shooting dope, the veins in my arm were bulbous and easy to find. Today they are sunken back and afraid of more punishment. It takes a few minutes of poking around, but finally I hit a vein. I know this because when I pull back to test, a rush of blood floods into the syringe and mixes with my fix. Knowing I'm there is almost a better high than actually pushing off. Once my thumb presses the plunger and the needle delivers, all my problems immediately disappear. In that moment, it doesn't matter how lonely I feel, how ashamed I am, how much money I owe, how many loved ones I've screwed over. I feel at peace.

Outside Looking In

Heroin addiction was never my problem. It was only a symptom. Drugs gave me the tranquility and serenity that I could never find on my own. I've always wanted to be comfortable in my own skin but didn't know how to get there. My deep-seated fears and insecurities seemed to always win out. Was I born insecure and afraid? Doubtful. I often try to examine, though, where my path went afoul.

When I was 14 years old, I had the best group of friends. We were rebels and misfits and it was the most fun of times. We graffitied, smoked weed, and went everywhere together. I don't remember being overly self-aware or uncomfortable back then. I felt part of something. Our crew had a name: DMT, an abbreviation for Demented. I would tag that name on every wall I could find and doodle it on every piece of paper I owned. I was a DMTer for life! At least, so I thought.

One day I got a call from the crew, not just one member but all of them, on speakerphone no less. They had apparently called a meeting that I was not a part of. The meeting was about me, and they unanimously decided to kick me out of Demented. These were all of my best friends and they were telling me what?! That I could no longer hang out with any of them? That the group I felt so close to and bonded with was giving me an unceremonious exit? I didn't see it coming. When I asked them why they did it, I couldn't get a logical answer. One by one, they just kept saying, "You need to make new friends." But I didn't want to. I thought I already had the best group of friends. They obviously didn't reciprocate that feeling. In ninth grade, it wasn't too easy to make new friends at a big high school. My only friend was my 12-year-old neighbor. When people in my class heard that I had but one friend and that he was a seventh grader, they laughed at me. This was the beginning of a lot of internal pain. I felt rejected and left out. At a time when the building blocks of social interaction were being formed for us freshmen, I was on the outside looking in. In my young mind, this event formed a strong pain memory that would last a very long time.

Pushing Through

The trauma of being shunned by my peers left me feeling hesitant and anxious in social situations. Eventually I made new friends and found a group that I could be a part of. Deep down, though, I was afraid that I wasn't really ever going to be a part of anything. I started doing more drugs and exploring new ways to act out. The more I could change the way I felt inside, the easier life was for me.

My journey through drug addiction spanned many years with plenty of high points but mostly low ones. It culminated when I was 19 years old with a year in LA County jail and no more bridges to burn. Unlike many of the people I used drugs with along the way, I was fortunate enough to get clean. To this, I credit the twelve steps and the many fellow addicts who have helped me over the years. Getting clean, however, was not the solution because the problem was never drugs. The problem was me. I only used heroin so I could escape my fears and uneasiness. As soon as the needle was taken away, I was faced with the reality of my situation. I was a young man with absolutely no idea of how to deal with life on life's terms.

From One Addiction to Another

Since childhood, one thing that has always given me comfort and solace is food. A great meal can conjure up the feelings of love and warmth that my mother gave me with her home-cooking. A full belly can make the emptiness and loneliness inside disappear for an instant. When I got clean and drugs were no longer an option for dealing with my problems, food became an easy solution. I loved the nod from a good shot in the arm. Just as much, I love the buzz from eating a savory meal. There is something so sensual about how food makes me feel. It transports me to a place of joy and satisfaction.

As I continued on my journey of sobriety, my relationship with food morphed into an unhealthy one. My addictive behavior transferred to how I ate. Binge eating become more frequent, but it was embarrassing so I started to hide it. Ordering two entrées at dinner with friends would elicit strange reactions, so I'd eat normally with them and get fast food by myself on the way home. My mind started to become increasingly preoccupied with what I was going to eat for the next meal, and I began making deals with myself about food: justifying binges by promising a juice fast in the near future.

Food wasn't the only vice I turned to when I got sober. Things like sex, love, validation, and shopping are all quick fixes. When I'm feeling empty or down, my mind can easily justify using a superficial remedy to feel better. But my relationship with the things that make me happy is always challenging. It's a fine line to walk, because I always crave more. Unfortunately, chasing good feelings isn't sustainable.

At the core lies the fear that I'm not enough, that I'm not loved, and that something is wrong with me. And none of these fears is addressed when I overeat, have a night of passionate sex with a new partner, or buy the latest smartphone. As soon as the food is eaten, my bed is empty, or my toys lose their cool, my mind tumbles down a whirlwind path of negative self-talk and I feel like the biggest piece of shit to ever walk this planet. Amidst this diseased thinking, I refute my own reality. I went to a gifted school as a child, but I believe I'm stupid. I have people who love me, but I believe I'm alone. I have money in the bank and a successful career, but I believe I'm a failure. And while it's not true, I believe that I'm fat and ugly.

I can talk myself into a reality of my own making where I'm worthless, and *this* is the crux of my problem. Food, sex, and shopping are temporary and superficial fixes, and eventually I had to find something in my recovery that would give me true harmony and peace.

Enter: Yoga

I am easily put off by anything hokey, so I rejected even the notion of yoga. Although I'd heard and read of the spiritual benefits of the practice, it seemed a little too kumbaya for my taste. I didn't think that it had anything to offer me—neither physically nor mentally / emotionally. Nevertheless, when I got out of jail at 20 years old, some old friends from high school were intent on dragging me to their favorite yoga studio. I resisted mightily, afraid of the tie-dyed and tofu-eating cult that I thought would be contorting their bodies next to mine. Yet my pals were relentless and eventually I gave in—if anything, simply to assuage their desire.

After my first-ever yoga class, my life was not changed. I didn't see God or make any grand proclamations about the new direction I would be embarking on. To be honest, it just felt good, surprisingly good. Yoga wasn't as new-agey as I thought it would be, and it seemed like a healthy tool to add to my life at the time. For a few years, I practiced once or twice a week and enjoyed the physical benefits the practice gave me.

But somewhere along the road, I decided to jump into yoga wholeheartedly and began to practice almost every day. I finally got what people were talking about when they mentioned that yoga was more than just physical. I started noticing that I was calmer in my life, that I was more present. Not only was I getting stronger and more open physically, but I was becoming clearer and less reactive mentally. My practice was no longer just about the poses but about *how* I was practicing them.

I was fortunate to have some great teachers teach me that yoga is a mind-body experience. Once I realized that, my time on the mat became much more powerful. It allowed me to be more conscious of my experience and be more aware of the truth. And, instead of being a prisoner of that truth, I now could wield my mind in a way to begin to change it. The benefits of the practice are simple and straightforward. Yoga did not magically and instantaneously remove my fears and insecurities. What it did do, though, is give me a little bit more strength to face them on a daily basis. Every morning I can make conscious choices of how to deal with my problems. It is completely up to me whether or not I choose to use the tools I've learned in my practice.

Transferred to the Body

When I wake up and get out of bed, I walk by my closet, which has a full-length mirror attached to it. Of course, because I'm incapable of not looking, I check out my naked body as I stroll past. Where does my mind go? It immediately goes to the parts of my body that I don't like. My belly: it's too big. My shoulders: not broad enough. My arms: not muscular enough. My face: ugly. My penis: small. Like a ritual, this happens every morning. I can't remember the first time that I hated my body, but I know it's been a while. Was it the media I was exposed to touting an unattainable standard of male beauty? Was it growing up among the über-narcissistic LA entertainment offspring? Was it those girls I heard gossiping in eighth grade about which guys were ugly and which were cute?

I may not know how my body image issues came to be, but I know why they still linger. It is a direct byproduct of the fear and insecurity I've been carrying around all these years, and no amount of external validation can fix that. No matter how many women (or men) tell me that I'm attractive, my default setting is that I'm ugly. No matter how many people mention how skinny I am, my default setting is that I'm fat. No matter how many partners rave about the caliber of my penis, it's tiny.

My distorted body image is so fixed, it won't let other people change my mind. I think they're just being nice and when they go home at night, they don't really believe the things they said. The solution has to come from within. How can I, using this same twisted mind that tells me the worst possible things about me, convince myself otherwise? How do I begin to walk through the fear and insecurity that have been plaguing me for so many years?

Small Shifts

It starts with my yoga practice. Since yoga introduced me to meditation, I consider meditation my yoga as well. One thing I've noticed is if I sit down first thing in the morning and take as few as five minutes to meditate before I begin my day, I'm better off. Sure, when I walk by the mirror, the negative self-talk is still there, but instead of rolling in that self-hatred, I can be present and conscious enough to pull myself out of it. It's not that the insecurities vanished, but I can focus my attention and energy where I choose. If I want to be happy, I redirect my focus on something positive. When I don't meditate in the morning, I don't have as much control over it and thus my peace of mind is a crapshoot.

My yoga practice has evolved over the last thirteen years, and I have become a yoga teacher, sharing the practice with others for eight years. I've found through teaching that sharing my personal experience can help others. I have never related to people preaching from a high horse, but I can always relate to those who've gone through similar experiences. That's why I'm sharing my story.

Because I am a yoga teacher, people perceive me as healthy, fit, and in a constant state of nirvana. Well, I'm a work in progress just like anyone else. Lots of students regularly ask me all kinds of life questions and requests for advice. Sometimes I'll even get asked about the same issues that I continue to struggle with. I think it's important for my students to know that I'm not any better than them. I have my demons too and I am far from perfect. The fears and insecurities that have plagued me since I was a teenager still come back into my consciousness regularly. My spiritual fitness is based on my consistent use of the tools I've learned.

No Finish Line

Since I began practicing yoga, it has grown from a small community into a worldwide one. For better or worse, yoga is part of mainstream culture and business is booming. The more people who practice yoga, the better off our planet will be, right? For the most part, I agree. However, there are pitfalls.

With mainstream business comes mainstream advertising. I can pull out the latest issue of a yoga magazine, see the beautiful, perfectly Photoshopped bodies in the ads, and go immediately into negative self-talk. As our yoga community grows and the yoga industry grows with it, there will be a steady increase of digitally altered and unattainable "perfection" depicted in yoga advertising, and I don't like what it brings into the yoga world.

For me, and for many I know, yoga has nothing to do with reaching a certain ideal. There is no finish line. There isn't one pose that will give me enlightenment, nor is there any sort of physical model that I am striving for. The physical practice is there for me to be strong, flexible, and healthy in a balanced and personal way. However, when I see those quintessential yoga pictures in ads, it is easy for me to feel I don't measure up, and I know a lot of other men who feel the same way I do. It isn't only women who have body image issues. Guys wrestle with the same worries that women do, except instead of our butts and legs, we worry more about our abs and arms.

While the changes to the culture of yoga that come with commodification aren't necessarily helping us, they are, however, allowing us to have this conversation. We do not practice yoga in a bubble. Whether or not the commercialization of yoga is here to stay, the issues will still be at hand. I get bombarded with ads to show me notions of perfection no matter where I go. Capitalism only works on the premise that we are not enough and need some product or service to find wholeness. Whether or not yoga businesses choose to use this model, pretty much every other business does.

How will I compare myself to the men that I see idealized in commercials? It is a difficult task to not feed into the misinformation that is perpetuated thousands of times per day. My yoga practice allows me to make choices. I don't have to be like those guys on the billboards to be happy. I can choose to be happy being me. It sounds cliché and easy, but for those of us who combat our negative self-image every day, we know that it is not. It takes vigilant practice, and yoga facilitates that.

Every moment of every day, I have a choice. Sometimes I choose to be positive and accepting of exactly who I am. Other times, I fall into the uneasy place of lacking and wanting. Being on the path for almost fifteen years now doesn't make me any more enlightened today than someone who maybe hasn't been practicing for that long. The reprieve that we are offered from yoga, meditation, and practicing principles is only a daily one. I can't stay clean from yesterday's shower, and in that same sense, I can't be positive from the mental space I was in twenty-four hours ago. Day by day and moment to moment, my mind fluctuates. It can take me to a bad place or a good one.

What I have learned from my time on this journey is that I have a choice. I can choose to be happy today, if I want. Most days I do. Some days I don't. It's progress, not perfection, and with each conscious choice I make, I get better at it. What helps me is remembering simple truths. In the end, will people really remember me for my abs? Or will people remember me for my positive and giving spirit? Today I try my best to put more energy in working toward the latter, for that is what makes me feel the best.

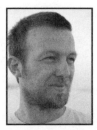

Vytas Baskauskas discovered a profound connection to yoga after a battle with addiction landed him in jail. What began as a form of therapy evolved into a way of life and a highly developed practice that he now shares with others as one of LA's premiere yoga instructors. He teaches at Yoga Works and Power Yoga East in Santa Monica, California, and is a professor of mathematics at Santa Monica College. www.VytasYoga.com

Author photo courtesy of the author.

CONFESSIONS OF A FAT, BLACK YOGA TEACHER

Dianne Bondy

*"My mission in life is not merely to survive,
but to thrive; and to do so with some passion,
some compassion, some humor, and some style."*—Maya Angelou

I am a fat, black yoga teacher. Yeah, I said it! Being called fat can be worse than a racial slur. I've had to endure both, and what saved me was yoga.

Society sets an impossible standard to live up to. Like most women, my struggles with weight and body image started young, and I have struggled with these issues most of my life. I've been really thin and fit, really thin and unfit, and I've been really fat and fit. I have also just been fat. I've done it all. Not long after my eighth birthday, I started gaining weight. Much to my parent's horror, I was becoming fat. In their eyes, nothing could be worse than being fat. My father especially hated it, and he thought he could shame me into being thin. He took every opportunity to humiliate and taunt me about my weight. He actually pulled me aside when I was about 10 years old and made a point of telling me I was a disappointment because I was fat and he'd never wanted a fat daughter. He relentlessly teased me in front of friends, family, and strangers.

On rare occasions he tried to be a decent father, but the biggest lesson he taught me was to be ashamed of myself. I think a lot of what he was trying to teach me was that being different was going to be a big challenge, and adding fatness to the mix would be a death sentence in modern society. A lasting lesson I learned from my dad was that I already had two strikes against me: I was black and a woman. The world would be cruel and discriminating based on these facts alone (let alone being fat). Being brown in a white world was going to be more than challenging, it was going to be daunting. It was something I could overcome; I just needed to be better than my best white counterpart to be considered worthy in this life. His words did not discourage me, though. Rather, they inspired me to be the best and to show the world that I would not, and cannot, live a mediocre life. Little did I know that yoga was going to be the vehicle that led down a path of great fulfillment and self-awareness!

No Charlie's Angel

I grew up in Burlington, Ontario, a small town in Canada. (We called it Borington.) Growing up in one of the only black families in our neighborhood added to my feelings of insecurity and isolation. Everywhere you went you stuck out like a sore thumb or a big brown spot in the middle of a sea of white faces. Everyone knew who you were and what your family did. We were an interesting oddity to everyone. Today, we would have our own reality TV show.

The standard of beauty back then was one of blue eyes, blond hair, and thin bodies. I think of Farrah Fawcett and *Charlie's Angels* when I think of the seventies and eighties. As a young black girl, I couldn't relate to anything I saw on TV, in movies, or in magazines. Being different was the kiss of death growing up as a brown girl in primary and middle school, and I had very few role models. One of them was my mom, and we had yoga.

Mother/Daughter Bonding Time

It took finding yoga and developing a serious practice to start changing the way I felt about myself. When I started, though, I was still miles away from understanding that. My mother introduced me to yoga when I was about 3. She'd just had twins. She had her hands full and couldn't leave the house. She had a book called *Stay Young with Yoga* (it was written in the 1950s and had funny pictures in it that fascinated me). There were no yoga or fitness models at this time, so it was just regular folks doing bendy things. This was my special mommy-and-me time when my brother and sister were napping.

My mom kept her yoga practice a secret. It was a time when yoga was the anti-culture—especially for people of color, who felt that yoga was something to be feared. A lot of black culture is steeped in deep religious beliefs, and it's a sin to question or run counter to the teachings of your pastor. Many religious leaders at that time (and some still today) within the black community felt that yoga is a vehicle of evil. However, my yoga practice has taught me that yoga only makes your beliefs stronger. My mom reminded me that yoga was my own special practice and that was all that was important. "Just enjoy breathing, practicing, and taking time," she would say.

Although I practiced next to my mother as a child, it was many more years before I fully began my journey with yoga. In high school and university, I fell into and out of many things designed to keep me skinny. I ran marathons, competed in fitness competitions, and taught hundreds of group fitness classes. These were distractions that kept my eating disorders and body image issues hidden. I thought that if I conquered my weight, I could conquer my feelings of inadequacy. Thus I ran on the hamster wheel of an unfulfilled life for years.

What Oprah Taught Me

I was taught that "Education is the greatest equalizer in modern times," and I truly believed that. Education is an investment in self—much like yoga is. I chose a university far from where I grew up. I saw it as a chance to reinvent myself. I could go somewhere no one knew me and become anyone. I could leave behind the fat, black kid. I went away to university in Windsor, Ontario. I was so excited to be right across the river from a predominately black city and to be so close to a culture I longed to be a part of. It was uplifting to feel like I fit in, and when I stepped on the university campus, I was excited to be part of something great. I thought that a higher education was going to solve all my problems. People here were going to be mature and accepting, I just knew it. I had arrived for the best part of my life … or so I thought.

In my quest to be part of the group at university, I was reminded again that black folks did not do yoga. So I gave up my yoga practice, succumbing to the pressure of wanting to fit in. I did it because for the first time in my life, I wasn't the only black person in the classroom and had the *opportunity* to fit in. I was in heaven, and I dove into black culture and enjoyed finally being part of a group.

I slowly learned, however, that giving up my practice didn't make me happy, and I felt it was time to challenge the idea that black people didn't do yoga! The catalyst for changing my mind about what people of color did was, yes, Oprah. I know it sounds cliché, but it's the truth. She's a pioneer, and she challenged people of color to think outside the box constructed by the dictates of society and religion. Oprah spoke like a yogi, and her personal philosophy appealed to me. She did things publicly that other people of color didn't do, and she was loved for it. Oprah proved that people of color can do anything. I picked up that torch and ran with it.

Yoga Studio or High School?

When I began to immerse myself back in my yoga practice, I took classes at a number of studios. I believed yoga culture would be open and accepting. I was nervous, but I was confident that I would be welcomed. What I found instead is that I still felt woefully out of place.

Once again, I didn't fit in. In fact, I often felt that I was back to square one: the big, fat, black blob in the sea of thin, young, white faces. It felt like high school all over again with judgment, cliquey groups, and exclusion. I sensed an underlying feeling of judgment as I stepped into each space. My big body belied my abilities. A fat yogi—how is this possible?

I distinctly remember going to an Ashtanga class and not being able to keep up because the "Ashtanga" I was practicing was really vinyasa, and I was confused. The teacher made comments throughout the practice that were diminishing to my spirit. She didn't call me out directly, but it was known to the class that I was distracting and not welcome back.

It was this feeling of exclusion that got me thinking I needed to open my own space. I started doing some recon work, and I continued to practice at many of the studios and gyms in my city, quietly observing what I didn't like and vowing to change it once I had my own space. I prayed and asked the powers that be for guidance, and my local church became my first yoga studio. The minister at my church felt that yoga would bring more people to church, and she supported my classes.

Being the Change

I put my intentions out there, and my classes grew. I made sure I taught to the people in the room, letting everyone know they could do it! The community at large embraced my message. I grew yoga from the small church hall into a full-time space. People would come through my doors from all different walks of life, including rolling in on wheelchairs, and they were welcomed. Our studio is known for its acceptance of diversity and its love of new students beginning the practice. To this day, people comment on what a welcoming space it is. It was this gift from my community that helped me open my heart to the idea that I was good enough to be a studio owner. I became the change I wanted to see in the studio.

Today yoga is becoming a lot more diverse. Speaking my mind and being seen in the yoga community has allowed me to connect to hundreds of people who practice yoga even though they aren't always the ones we see in the media. People of all shapes, sizes, ages, abilities, class backgrounds, and shades practice yoga.

Most of my experiences in yoga have been restricted to my city. After years of training and teaching, I decided to step out of my comfort zone and head to Tucson to study yoga with some of the most advanced yoga teachers in the world. Once again, though, I was the only bigger-bodied black girl in the room. It was a devastating week spent openly crying on my mat in front of sixty advanced yoga students. I felt so lost. I'd dragged my family thousands of miles for what? I begged my husband to go home, and he told me I had to go back and face the music on my mat. Clearly, it was something I needed to work through, and it became a turning point for me. It made me realize that I can't be only one who feels so lost.

That week taught me that doing advanced arm balances didn't have to be my thing. It also taught me that I needed to create a diverse yoga space, help grow diverse teachers, and do my part in making yoga more accessible. I am tired of workshops and training where teachers say not everyone will be able to do this pose so some of you will have to watch. WHAT?! Inflexible people should not be mere spectators, paying money for workshops where they just watch the flexible doing yoga.

When I opened my feelings globally through writing about my experiences, others reached out to me and shared similar feelings about their yoga practices. I found that curvy-bodied teachers, teachers of color, teachers with varying gender identities and expressions, and students of all walks of life were united in the cause of expanding everyone's perception of yoga, a practice that should be accessible to every body. It's these connections that helped me refine my voice and gave me courage to move forward with my mission in yoga and diversity.

You Teach Yoga?

I'm always nervous when I head into a new venue to teach yoga. There was a time when I was also a little bit scared of being an imposter because I didn't fit the yoga stereotype. When I enter a space, I am often met with the same reaction: *"You* teach yoga?" I usually get a once-over, and the judgment in their eyes is palpable.

I recently hosted a retreat at a beautiful yoga resort in Aruba. It just so happened that the owner of that spectacular retreat space was down for the week on his monthly visit to inspect the property. I was introduced to him, and I recognized "the look" right away when he asked twice if *I* was teaching the retreat. I noticed it again when it came time to teach and he began closely observing me. My teaching skills seemed to surprise him, and he praised my abilities. Why is it so shocking that a big person could be a halfway decent yoga teacher?

How do we shake up the yoga stereotypes and allow people to see yoga as it really is? We are not all white, able-bodied, super-flexible, thin, heterosexual beings. We are diverse in every way and it's this diversity that makes life interesting.

We can change the misperception of what yoga looks like by encouraging people to become stewards of their own wellness. They don't need external validation—they can find what they are looking for within themselves. And yoga can help them find it. They shouldn't feel like they need permission to practice. Yoga is a vehicle to wellness; it's about the mind-body-spirit connection. We don't need to fit into these narrow yoga stereotypes to practice yoga. We must encourage people who feel marginalized and who are different that we need their uniqueness and experiences. We need to develop a conscious culture committed to social justice and equality for every body.

Turning Inward

Yoga is all about the breath, quieting the mind, and tuning into your true nature. The *asana* (or yoga pose) portion of yoga is discussed as the third limb in Patanjali's sutras, which leads me to believe that it isn't the most important part of the practice, but one of many equally important parts.

When we fail to offer modifications to struggling students, we create an exclusive club of the cans and cannots. The cans may have the unfair advantages or privileges, namely genetics and sometimes even a gymnastics background. The cannots may be (note: this doesn't fit with the theme of body modifications) older, tighter, or bigger bodied. Unfortunately, most yoga studios today don't include the cannots, and here lies the problem. It already occurs in everyday society, and now we've allowed this to steep into our spiritual and wellness practices. Yoga is about what you can do, not what you cannot do.

Making Changes

How do you make your teacher trainings, workshops, and events accessible for everyone involved? You learn how to teach inclusively. My motto is "No Yogi Left Behind." There is a place for everyone on the mat; we just have to change our mindset.

The key to bringing diversity to yoga is to have a diversity of teachers. Inclusion on the yoga mat means everyone is welcome—to teach and practice. How do you get bigger people to go to yoga classes? Have more bigger-bodied teachers. How do you get a more culturally diverse yoga class? You train culturally diverse yoga teachers to teach. We need to learn how to teach progressively so that students of varying abilities and experience levels can practice in the same room safely and comfortably.

We also need to be more inclusive and sensitive in how we speak. Language is powerful. When we hear the term "diversity," most of us automatically think of people of color. But diversity exists on many levels. We are diverse within our cultures, our bodies, and our beliefs. Diversity refers to different socioeconomic classes, ages, races, genders, sexual orientations, and sizes. And yoga should be accessible to everyone in this diversity. In fact, it should be celebrated in all yoga classes.

Yoga studio owners and teachers need to offer classes that are truly accessible to every body—no matter that body's size, age, level of flexibility, strength, or ability.

Every *asana* has a modification, and teachers should offer those modifications to their students. Teachers should make students aware that the person who is concentrating on their breathing, listening to their body, finding the version of the pose that they need, or taking breaks is "doing" yoga perfectly. And that they shouldn't compare themselves to the person who is in the most advanced version of the pose. Completing an advanced version of a pose doesn't make that person a better yogi. There is no better or worse in yoga.

Those of us who are different need to find, connect with, and support each other. We need to set aside the idea that we can't just show up to the mat as ourselves. The people who are going to judge us based on our size, color, gender, or physical challenges are not truly practicing yoga.

My challenge to you is to change the culture, change the language, and change the idea of what yoga teachers and yoga students look like. Be a trailblazer. Share your uniqueness, your challenges, and your practice.

You have something powerful to offer the world.

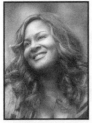

Dianne Bondy is the founder of Yogasteya, an online yoga studio that caters to people of all shapes, sizes, and ethnic and cultural backgrounds. As a studio owner, full-time yoga teacher, writer, and public speaker, Dianne is passionate about empowering people to realize their full potential on and off the mat. www.yogasteya.com
Author photo by Erika Reid.

I'M A WARRIOR, HEAR ME ROAR

Carrie Barrepski

I have always thought of my disabilities as characteristics. Having cerebral palsy, congenital heart disease, and being hearing impaired and legally blind does not define who I am. From an early age, I was never afraid to try anything new, from ballet to playing the guitar. Even though there were difficulties, I have enjoyed every single minute of the experience. Life is full of challenges and obstacles that can be overcome with the right attitude and hard work. I have always been strong-willed and determined. One of my husband's favorite quotes from Steve Jobs's biography says it all. Bill Atkinson, an Apple engineer, reflecting on one of his breakthroughs in the Apple II / very early Mac days, said, "Because I didn't know it couldn't be done, I was enabled to do it." I have always believed that there is a solution to every problem as long as you believe in it. The key is to never give up and keep on trying until you get it right.

Support and Challenges

I was very fortunate in my childhood to have the best parents possible and the most fun sister in the world, who made my childhood very enjoyable. I also formed one of the longest, best friendships of my life with Shannon, the girl next door. Even though we later went through years of separation, we always managed to find each other and keep our friendship intact. I feel thankful that I had a good support system with family and friends.

I have developed many tools and learned many lessons from my experiences with disabilities. The most important one was to learn how to be a strong advocate. After graduating from high school, I went from having teachers take care of all of my accessibility needs to having to do it all on my own, such as finding my own note takers in college, explaining my disabilities to my professors, and getting documents enlarged. I also learned how to use my voice to express my concerns and needs in a productive way. In addition, I acquired compassion for people in similar situations, and I am always willing to help.

I faced many obstacles in my high school and college years. One of them was that a high school guidance counselor told me I should not bother applying to colleges due to low SAT scores. At first I was devastated, but my teaching consultant, Terry Leaga, counseled me that SAT scores were not the only things that colleges looked at; they also considered factors such as GPA and individual characteristics. Another challenge that occurred in high school was that I had to deal with an ignorant teacher who did not want a disabled student in his class. For instance, he faced the chalkboard while talking, refused to give me materials to be enlarged, and made me feel unwelcome. He was reprimanded and had to deal with me in his class. Despite his behavior, I passed his class with high grades. During my college years, I had to prove myself over and over again. However, in all, I loved my college years, and it is there that I met one of my best friends, Danielle.

Soul Mates

The most important relationship that I have developed in my life is with my husband, Frank. I found it difficult to meet people because I was being judged by my disabilities rather than my character. One night, in an online hearing loss chat room, I met a fellow chatter with a hearing loss. Frank had gotten a cochlear implant in 1997, and we had similar experiences with our hearing loss. In classes, Frank often used an FM system for the deaf, which is essentially a miniature radio station in which a microphone worn by the professor transmits the sound to the person wearing a receiver that amplifies the sound for that person.

Frank has had his own challenges with his hearing loss. One experience he had was with a college professor who didn't want to use the microphone for the FM system. After the school's Disability Services Office was informed of this, the professor was ordered to wear the microphone. However, a relationship grew between Frank and the professor to the point where at the end of the class Frank was asked to be a teaching assistant for that class the next semester, which he continued doing for most of his years there.

We soon discovered that we had similarities from our childhoods and family life. Both of our fathers were insurance fraud investigators and both passed away while we were in college. We each have one older sister. We are both bookworms and love computers. Our bond grew stronger over the two years that we chatted until we decided to meet in May 2004. At that time, Frank flew from Massachusetts to Michigan to meet me. We then flew back and forth visiting each other, and by Thanksgiving 2004 we were engaged to be married. In June 2005, we were married surrounded by family and friends. Due to Frank's law practice, I moved to Massachusetts and built up my freelance writing career. I have been very fortunate to grow a strong, loving relationship with my in-laws, who became my second family. As of this writing, we have been married eight years and counting.

My Yoga Background

All the support I had, in addition to my own determination, encouraged me to try many things. In my late 20s, I began looking for an exercise program that would meet my needs. I chose yoga because somebody told me it was good for stiff muscles and flexibility. I tried several yoga DVDs, but I felt intimidated by many of the advanced yoga poses. Then I discovered Seane Corn's DVDs, *Vinyasa Flow Yoga: Uniting Movement and Breath*. It was Seane's instructions and modifications of yoga poses that helped me fall in love with the practice, and soon I was doing it every day.

In my practice I use yoga props such as blocks and straps to modify yoga poses. Seane herself demonstrated many of these options. I also experimented with my practice, coming up with my own variations of yoga poses. I came to trust and listen to my body's cues on what it can and cannot do. For example, in many of the floor exercises, such as the forward bend, I use a yoga strap. The yoga block is useful for doing poses such as Downward-Facing Dog.

I have kept up my morning practice with Seane, along with getting to know her through e-mail, Facebook, and workshops. She has become a mentor in my daily practice and work. After years of doing DVDs by myself, I felt brave enough to try a yoga class.

I remember being nervous because I make a lot of modifications to poses. When I arrived at the yoga class, I spoke with the teacher about my physical limitations and making my own modifications. He reassured me that I would be fine and to just take my time. I felt connected with the other students, and I was relieved to see that I was not the only one who needed to make modifications.

At the conclusion of the class, the teacher told me he was impressed with how I took care of myself and listened to my body. After being in the class, I realized each person's practice is their own and yoga is about being mindful of what's happening to your body. This mindfulness can be carried out in our daily life, in our eating, our words, and our actions. During a class at Kripalu Center, the teacher said: "Our yoga mat is our science lab because we are experimenting with our body movements." I remember this when I am doing yoga; it is so true since our bodies move in different ways.

Off the Mat

One day I picked up a yoga magazine featuring Seane, who talked about spiritual activism in taking yoga off the mat into your daily life. This came at a time when I didn't know what I wanted to do with my life, since I was unable to find a social work job that did not require a driver's license, and I was stuck in a dead-end job at a department store. Seane's words inspired me to turn my passions for writing and helping people with disabilities into my purpose.

I started writing for several online disability websites. Eventually, I wrote a monthly column called "Disability Talks" in my hometown paper, and I now have a weekly column. My platform for my work is to empower people with disabilities to be independent and advocate for themselves. I encourage individuals to focus on their strengths and talents while working on strengthening their weaknesses. I have written on many issues, such as laws, discrimination, health concerns, and coping with everyday life. I have also had the opportunity to speak to organizations on a variety of topics from advocacy to living with disabilities. I believe we each have a voice that deserves to be heard. I received an award for my work as a disability rights advocate from the Stavros Center for Independent Living.

One of my proudest accomplishments has been working on a project called the Wheel Walk. Stanley Park has been dedicated to making its park accessible for people with disabilities, such as having an adaptive walking trail and an ADA-accessible playground. Every summer a group of advocates, including myself, come together to bring awareness to accessibility in the park with activities that include a walkathon and a barbecue.

Yoga has helped me determine my passion and purpose as a writer and activist dedicated to helping to inspire people with disabilities. I will continue to do this by using my voice in love, passion, and compassion to make a difference.

My Body Image

I have struggled with my body image from having a hump in my back, curved shoulders, and a different-looking body. Shopping for clothing has been a challenge for me, especially dresses. After becoming engaged, I was confronted with the scary task of finding a wedding dress. I was petrified that I would not find a dress that fit properly. I remember pulling up to David's Bridal Shop with my mother, who gave me the advice just to go in and have fun by trying on different dresses. Behold, the first dress I tried on was absolutely perfect. Both my mother and sister assured me that I looked beautiful and that this was going to be my wedding dress. Sometimes when you let go of your fears, things have a way of working out. I had feelings of shame and wanted to look like everyone else. The funny part of this is that in my work, I am always talking about how we are all beautiful, unique people inside and outside, and you would think I would take my own advice.

Since my childhood, my mother encouraged me to keep a journal. She would say that after writing down the negatives, turn the page and start fresh. This was her way of saying to let go of the negativity and focus on the positive. My parents taught my sister and me to never compare ourselves to each other because we are each our own person. I feel this is probably one of the most valuable lessons I have ever learned. It is something that I express in both my personal and professional lives, along with the importance of being independent.

Today, I am still working on my body image and learning to follow my own advice to accept yourself for who you are. I am also learning that being healthy is an important part of body image, from eating healthy to exercising. I treat my body as a temple because we each have just one body to take care of.

Today I depend on my daily yoga practice with Seane Corn and Ashley Turner to keep me fit and balanced. My yoga practice along with Pilates always leaves me feeling healthy. I have also developed a strong spiritual and meditation practice with the help of Gabrielle Bernstein's books. These practices keep me focused and positive every day. I follow a semi-vegetarian diet filled with fruits, vegetables, whole grains, and beans. I believe in eating in moderation and being mindful of what you put into your body—and that everybody deserves a small treat once in a while.

Health Challenges

In the spring of 2012, I was diagnosed with a leaky heart valve. My cardiologist told me the best treatment would be heart surgery to replace the valve. This was a reminder to me how important and precious our health is. After I had the surgery, I depended on my meditation and visual imagination to help deal with pain, fears, and frustration. I was also very blessed to have supportive family and friends who supported and encouraged me to get healthy. I soon learned the value of resting during my recovery. Today I still take time out during the day to rest. That experience has empowered me to put my health first while improving on my body image as a picture of good health.

Yoga is a valuable tool for dealing with negative self-talk. Combining meditation, deep breathing, and poses allows me to focus on the positive images while letting the negatives flow away. I am often reminded of a quote by one of my favorite yoga teachers, Kathryn Budig, who said, "Aim for your truth." I take this to mean that the practice of yoga allows you to zero in on who you really are and what your goals are.

When I look in the mirror, I see a strong, free-spirited person who is beautiful on the inside and outside. I have grown to love myself, to be proud of who I am and what I have accomplished.

Becoming a Yoga Teacher

As a yogi, my practice affects every part of my life and has become a way of life. One of my longtime goals was to share my yoga experience with others with limitations. That opportunity developed when I attended the Off the Mat Leadership Training Series at the Omega Yoga Center in Rhinebeck, New York. It was there, at the organization founded by my teacher, Seane, that I decided to make my goals into a reality. This training was all about sharing your yoga practice and philosophy, and that's just what I decided to do.

In the spring of 2013, I went through the Lakshmi Voelker chair yoga teacher training so I could help people with physical limitations such as mine enjoy the full benefits of yoga. Like me, Lakshmi believes everyone can do yoga. This training program was conducted over Skype, with Lakshmi's camera connected to our TV so the lessons would be easier with my visual impairment. I instantly fell in love with the classes, especially learning how to adapt poses to the chair, including Sun Salutations, balance poses, and the Warrior pose series. Now my favorite activity is to find new ways to adapt yoga to the chair.

When I taught my first class, I felt as I if I was being guided by my teachers to share my love of yoga with others. I spoke from my heart and my truth, empowering my students to feel the power of yoga. Some of my favorite feedback is that I have passion and love for the practice that is shared with everyone. Now that I am a teacher, I am much more aware of my self-image because I want to reflect positive feelings to my students. I want to practice what I teach, from self-love to healthy habits.

It thrills me to no end to be living out my passion and purpose of helping people with disabilities be independent and proud of who they are. I love sharing my experiences and inspiring people to be more active in their lives and communities. I am living my best life because I am able to combine my three passions of yoga, writing, and disability advocacy into one connective group. I am proud to be a wife, yogi, writer, teacher, and activist.

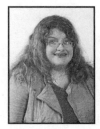

Carrie Barrepski is a disability rights activist and columnist writing about disability issues to help and inspire others. As a longtime yogini, she is a Lakshmi Voelker chair yoga teacher sharing the joy of yoga with those with physical limitations. www .carriewrites.net

Author photo courtesy of *The Republican*.

YOGA FROM THE MARGINS

Teo Drake

It's an ungodly hour on a Sunday morning and I am sweating.

Mind you, I don't do well with heat. Here I am in flannel pajamas dumbfounded in the midst of my very first attempt at yoga, trying to understand what I'm experiencing. Later I would learn that it was *chaturanga* and vinyasa flow, but in the moment it seems like I should be throwing my body at the ground at ninety miles an hour, which I have now tried to do four or five times, and all I've gotten for my troubles is a puddle of sweat.

I came to this moment having no idea what yoga was. It wasn't something that showed up in the working-class, Italian Catholic neighborhood I grew up in or in my family of factory workers and mail carriers and nurses. It wasn't something that showed up in my small-town queer social networks. I didn't come from places where there would have been an invitation to do yoga. I was far more likely to enter a martial arts studio—which I recently had done, in fact, and it was there that I was running into issues of inflexibility with the compact, muscle-bound, locked-down body that I brought.

People would occasionally tell me that yoga would help me relax or help me with flexibility, and because of this I think I thought that doing yoga meant relaxing, flopping around in shapes, maybe some meditating. I probably confused it a little with tai chi. So because I was thinking it was a relaxing activity and yoga is readily available online and on DVDs, eventually I decided I was willing to give it a try in the privacy of my own home, where I could potentially make a fool of myself and no one could see me. I'd already been to a martial arts studio and been thrown head over heels onto the mat. I'm thinking, "I got this!" with my cup of coffee and my flannel pajama pants on and my $9.99 yoga mat. How hard could it be?

But now, twenty minutes into my completely unexpected and not at all relaxing introduction to yoga, exhausted, in a puddle of sweat, I give up. I retreat into child's pose and refuse to come out except to once reach for my coffee mug, like a petulant child grasping for a safety blanket. Then I permanently go back to child's pose and won't be budged.

———

If you are thinking that surely this must have been both the beginning and the end of my relationship with yoga, I wouldn't be surprised. But the miracle in it all is that rather than give in to my wounded pride, I 'fessed up to my defeat to various folks in my life, a number of whom recommended that I check out a beginner's yoga class, and I was actually willing to give that a try.

The further miracle was that I found my way to a yoga studio located in an industrial district of oil suppliers and machinists, which meant it felt accessible to me in a way that so many mainstream, boutique yoga studios never would have. I am also grateful that I found myself in a gentle yoga class held in the middle of the day, attended by a handful of older folks, and taught by an amazing teacher who had found yoga later in life. A youthful, feisty woman in her 60s, she was a good, grounded, kind soul who taught from a really accessible place. She talked about her own limitations and created space for me and my fellow practitioners to talk about our bodies and where we struggled, and when she discussed ways of navigating all that, she did it from a matter-of-fact place rather than treating our bodily limitations as something to overcome.

And so my first yoga teacher modeled an embodied practice without having to leave a part of myself at the door or pathologize a part of who I was—all of me came to the mat and some parts of me moved differently than others and it was all part of the practice. She brought yoga alive for me from a place of understanding and negotiating bodies that weren't lithe and sinewy and inherently flexible. To this day I'm grateful for the joy, whimsy, and humor she brought to that imperfect practice.

It's important to understand what met me on the mat. What met me on the mat was a culmination of a lifetime of being at war with myself and of living in a culture that was at war with me. I had never been comfortable in my own body, and I had lived a lifetime of hearing messages that told me what I knew about myself couldn't be true and how I understood my body was wrong. As a survivor of childhood physical abuse, domestic violence, and addiction, as someone who at that point had been living with HIV/AIDS for twelve years, the idea of being more physically present in my body was like being asked to move to a war zone—a far more imaginable prospect. Truth be told, my body *was* a war zone. Around any corner there could be a minefield, and that corner could be the last one I turned, because I couldn't bear what I might find if I kept going.

I found yoga five years after I had started gender transition, and a few years after I'd had chest reconstruction surgery. It took the threat of dying young from AIDS for me to find the courage to transition from female to male; because now nothing was more frightening than dying, I could risk everything to live in authenticity. At the age of 38, my relationship to my body was new, as was the way other people interacted with me based on what they saw—when I first came to that gentle yoga class, I probably appeared to be an incredibly fit, muscled, and healthy man (although no one would have called me agile, that's for sure). The class started very slow, but even that was hard for me. I had never moved my body in that way before. I had never been attentive when my body moved. I had played softball, whitewater kayaked, I had been practicing martial arts for about a year, but I didn't have any ability to move with intention and be present. I moved from a place of reaction. And so those really slow movements were hard to do and stay present.

My body was tight and compact, inflexible to the point of snapping, and unfamiliar. Being present in my body was like going on a trip where someone else had packed my luggage. Every single time someone asked me to simply stand in Mountain pose, roll my shoulders back, and open my chest, I had to confront the fact that I couldn't do it—my muscles had constricted and my shoulders had rounded in response to physical violence and from decades of hiding my chest. I had to actively see, for the first time, all the ways I had turned in, curled up, locked down on a structural level. I had to experience the waves of agony and grief and loss that the simplest yoga movements brought forward for me.

———

From as young as I can remember, I hated myself. The violence at home only added confirmation that I was despised and disposable. The terror of the unpredictable violence was inextricable from the fear of knowing I was a boy but believing that to voice that truth would have been the last straw. The only way you can make sense of being beaten in a fit of rage as a little kid is to take it personally. The only power you have in those moments is to believe that it is happening because of something about you and if you could just change, it would stop. If I could just be a girl, if I could stop asking *why*, if I could stop embarrassing my parents, the violence would stop. But it never stopped.

I spent more than thirty-five years trying to die in all kinds of active and passive ways. I drank. I drank not to feel better, not to feel looser. I drank to die. One particular night, when I was hospitalized for alcohol poisoning, I was full of rage. Rage that I wasn't dead yet. I had made a serious effort, having consumed thirty shots of vodka in four hours. That deep agony just called out to be held. If only someone had wrapped their arms around my teenage self and rocked me. Instead I got strapped to a bed and lectured by a priest on how in my queerness I was aiding the devil's work.

My healing began in my early 20s when I entered twelve-step recovery. Somehow I could again hear that small voice that had spoken to me in childhood, that soft voice of the divine that told me I was loved and wanted, and this led me to seek a new spiritual path as a means of climbing out of the dark pit of despair that I had lived in for so long. From a grounding in twelve-step spirituality, I went on to find Buddhism. The idea of a spiritual practice rooted in compassion and kindness resonated deeply with me after a lifetime of isolation and anger. When yoga came into my life, it tied in so many of the spiritual principles of Buddhism and twelve-step work that it felt familiar. And when I heard yogis such as Seane Corn talk about embodied activism, and also about light and shadow, I felt like they were speaking my language. These yogis came from dark places but didn't hide that darkness, so when they said they were alive today because of yoga I could believe them.

The gift that gender transition offered me was the possibility that it could be safe to be physically present in my own body. What yoga offered me was an actual pathway to get there. Because of the way that trauma shows up for me in my body, my primary response is to freeze—I get locked down, I get numb, and I can't think clearly. Physically, emotionally, and cognitively, I can't move. Finding ways of being present, as someone who has all the reasons in the world to dissociate, was a huge task.

By experiencing discomfort in small, manageable ways on the mat and learning to breathe through it, yoga offered me a practical skill to deal with dissociation. The reality is that painful feelings were happening all the time, but no one taught me how to live with them. When it was so intolerable to be in my body and be present, all yoga asked of me was to breathe and move. And so I would get profoundly uncomfortable and I didn't have to make it okay. It didn't have to be pretty, because my life wasn't pretty. The idea that I could just breathe and move allowed me to start to unlock my frozenness. Until I started practicing yoga, I didn't understand that the path to healing was that simple and that hard.

Learning to be fluid in my body through a vinyasa flow practice, learning to be compassionate and gentle with my body, is really my spiritual and physical edge. I know how to be strong, locked down, tight, physically powerful—but being physically powerful and emotionally present is something I don't always know how to do. The physical unlocking of my body is still happening—my dense knotted back muscles can attest to the fact that I'm not "unlocked," just less locked down. But yoga and martial arts have helped my trauma-frozen self develop the ability to move and be fluid.

———

Over the years, my understanding of what it means to have a yoga practice has evolved, and my practice has included vinyasa flow, restorative practice, and the Bhakti practice of chanting. There have been periods of physical wellness where I have enjoyed four-days-a-week vinyasa flow classes, and there are times where all I can manage is breathing in child's pose. Living with AIDS means there are many times when my physical ability and my stamina are beyond my control. It's in those moments that I'm grateful for the early lessons I received that taught me yoga was about landing physically, spiritually, and emotionally in the same place, on my mat. If all I can manage is child's pose, that's yoga. If Bhakti chanting is where I'm at, that's yoga. If it serves to open my heart and my mind and my spirit and allows me to be compassionate with myself and with the world around me, that's yoga. I don't know if I'm ever truly going to not be at war with myself on some level. But I do know that yoga never fails to help me negotiate a gentle truce.

Every one of us has a relationship with our body that is negotiated; we just aren't all equally aware of it. Some of us are incredibly aware of it because we've had to have open negotiations with our bodies simply to survive. I happen to have a conscious understanding and a language for talking about this because I've had to examine my physical form in such a raw way. But I think we all do it. Some of us do it with greater intention than others. Some of us do it in ways that make us whole, and some of us do it in ways that tear us apart. For me, yoga was the one way I found to bring compassion into those negotiations with my body.

Because of this, I struggle with the lack of awareness in mainstream Western yoga culture about what it takes for so many of us to show up, about the sheer courage it takes to have that negotiation in a public space, and about what it takes to make spaces fully accessible to the huge numbers of people who will never feel comfortable coming in to your typical yoga studio.

Every time I enter a mainstream US yoga studio, I feel barraged by an emphasis on pretty spaces and pretty clothes and pretty bodies. I feel the weight of constant messaging that yoga is about incredibly complicated poses that only a certain percentage of bodies are ever going to be able to do. I am faced with the financial inaccessibility of memberships and cost-prohibitive drop-in classes, and the worse inaccessibility in terms of what it feels like to walk in with oil under my nails, work boots heavy and noisy on the polished floors, being greeted by the assumption that I must be new to yoga because I don't look like someone who practices yoga. And every time I have to struggle with whether there's a space that's physically safe for me to change in—nine times out of ten there's not. When I've approached studios about catering classes and spaces to queer and trans folks, I've had to hear, "Everyone's welcome! We don't need a separate class for queer and trans people." Yet I can't even get into my yoga clothes safely to make it to class.

If I somehow do navigate all of these obstacles, there's the equally difficult hurdle of trying to get into my body while facing a new onslaught of inaccessible language from the teacher. I'm hearing language about men's bodies and women's bodies that deny my existence. I'm hearing "if you're an advanced practitioner..." instead of "for those who want more sensation..." or "to move to another level..." If your next level is putting your legs behind your head and your thumbs in your ears and wiggling about on your butt cheeks, I'm all for it, but don't call that "advanced."

Because my advanced is that I'm here; I got through all of those personal and cultural barriers and showed up. I guarantee you that being in my body, as stiff and as rigid and as terrified as I am, and simply bending over and having a conversation with my toes from eight inches away is pretty damn advanced. If all that yoga represents is being able to fling your feet behind your head without requiring any emotional presence whatsoever, then we've taken yoga away from its true intent.

My deepest hope is that the voices from the margins—those who are practicing yoga and those who could be practicing yoga—will be heard as we continue to come forward and that the mainstream Western yoga community can adapt and change. What I don't want is the mainstream yoga world to make room for us, in its version of yoga. What I want is for our experiences to shape and shift how yoga is currently practiced. I want us to come back home to an understanding of yoga from a place of embodiment and service. I don't want to be invited to assimilate. What I want is a call and an invitation into a universal process of radical welcome and transformation.

———

Despite all of the healing that meditation, Buddhism, twelve-step recovery, and therapy utilizing somatic experiencing have brought me, to this day when I put my forehead to my mat in child's pose to begin my yoga practice, this is the only place where I ever feel truly physically present in my body, and as at home as I can ever get. Child's pose is the place I always go where I will without fail hear that loving soft voice of the divine, telling me that I am loved, that I am needed, that I am wanted.

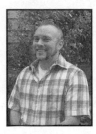

Teo Drake is a spiritual activist, an educator, a practicing Buddhist and yogi, and an artisan who works in wood and steel. He is affiliated with Off the Mat, Into the World and the organization Transfaith. When this blue-collar, queer-identified trans man living with AIDS isn't helping spiritual spaces be more welcoming and inclusive of queer and transgender people or helping queer and trans folks find authentic spiritual paths, he can be found teaching martial arts, yoga, and woodworking to children. www.rootsgrowthetree.com
Author photo courtesy of the author.

FROM BODY CONFIDENT
TO BODY INSECURE AND BACK

Joni Yung

I am a short, middle-aged, average-looking Asian woman … and I have somehow found myself lost in a sea of leggy 20-something aspiring-model blond yoginis. I'm finding it a bit hard to figure out where I belong.

Yes, I've had my share of self-image issues through the years, with the usual attempts to solve them. Crash diets. New Year's resolution gym memberships. Heavy investment in black wardrobe items.

I finally hopped off the hamster wheel over twenty years ago when I made health and fitness a permanent part of my lifestyle. Since then, I've taken thousands of yoga classes in over a hundred yoga studios, run at least fifty marathons in more states than most people have visited in their lifetimes, and have logged more miles by bike than I did by car last year. I've also adapted a pescetarian diet—or as I put it, I eat anything that doesn't have feet. So you'd probably assume that I'm physically fit, and that I'm confident with the way I look and who I am. And up until maybe five years ago, I would have agreed with you on all counts.

But thanks to yoga, my self-esteem has taken a serious nosedive.

My Early Carefree Days

Born in Los Angeles in the late fifties to Filipino parents, my earliest memories were of being the kid who didn't quite fit in—from being the only Asian kid in my kindergarten class to being the only kid who couldn't speak Tagalog in my second-grade class when my parents moved back to the Philippines.

But by the time I reached the third grade, I had pretty much blended in with the rest of my classmates; I looked, spoke, and acted like everyone else. The usual adolescent image insecurities soon followed: cokebottle glasses in the fifth grade, crooked teeth in the sixth, stubborn baby fat in the seventh, but all were resolved in the summer before high school when I got contact lenses, braces, and a painful case of mumps when I couldn't eat anything for a week. It's funny how Mother Nature knew how to give me what I wanted when I wanted it!

They say your teen years are the best years of your life. And I have to agree—I was able to eat everything in sight and you'd never know it, thanks to a raging metabolism that burned off all calories before I even ingested them. Ah, to be young again.

Up and Down the Diet Roller Coaster

After graduating with a computer science degree from UCLA, I entered the workforce in the late seventies as a programmer. After a handful of years planted in front of a computer screen, I realized my clothes no longer fit the way they used to. I joined a gym and soon was chanting the Jane Fonda no-pain-no-gain mantra, but all those aerobics classes soon got old and I stopped going. An extra five pounds crept back on, but there was no reason for me to obsess about them; I was gainfully employed and newly engaged to my longtime boyfriend. Life was good.

When it came time to buy a wedding dress, I decided that I didn't want to be remembered for all time as looking pudgy in my wedding photos, so I went on a crash diet and lost those five pounds by my wedding day. And promptly gained them back by the time we'd returned from our honeymoon a month later.

Being pregnant was a joy because not only was I morning sick-ness–free, but I truly believed that I was eating for two, which I did with gusto. I gained a whopping 45 pounds by the time I delivered my firstborn daughter. I lost most of it by her first birthday, just to put on another 40 during my second pregnancy. After a string of short-lived diet attempts—low fat, high protein, low carb, high fiber—I was still two dress sizes larger than I wanted to be. But my role as a working mother kept my mind on other things, so I eventually accepted my new rounded look.

Over lunch one day at the office, a coworker—and close friend—commented on how he'd noticed that I was fond of eating fried and sugar-laden food. How could I, as intelligent as I was, continue to eat stuff that would kill me? After all, my father had a stroke, my mother had gout, and both were diabetic; if I kept eating the way I had been, there was a good chance I'd end up with the same health problems as my parents. Yikes.

I cut down on fried food, ate more veggies, joined yet another gym, and within a year, I'd lost so much weight that I was thinner than I was on my wedding day. All I had to do was eat sensibly and exercise regu-larly, and the weight took care of itself. Genius!

The Weekend Warrior

I skipped work one day to go skiing with my healthy-living guardian angel and a mutual buddy. High on altitude and fast conditions, the two men decided on a whim to race each other at the upcoming LA Mara-thon. They turned to me: Would I be interested in upping my workout routine and training with them? I proclaimed them insane and instead bought a bike and rode alongside them for exercise as they ran up and down the beach path, mile after mile after mile.

It was great having a mentor to keep an eye on my eating and exercise habits—and my relapses—at the office, but the true test came a year later when I found myself leaving that job for another one. This time, I was on my own.

As fate would have it, I happened to make small conversation with a woman I'd met at the gym. Over one of the usual "who are you and what do you do for fun" conversations, she mentioned that she had just run her first marathon and that she was training to climb to the top of Mount Whitney. Whoa. This was from a slightly overweight woman whom I'd pegged as a couch potato? I took this as a challenge: if she could do it, so could I. Whitney's 14,505 foot peak was a bit too high for this acrophobe, so I opted to take on the sea-level road race instead. She ran with a marathon training group whose registration opened in a month. I knew that if I didn't act on it then, it would never happen.

Shock would be an understatement to describe the look on the faces of my marathon finisher friends when I told them about my latest endeavor. So to make sure I wouldn't wimp out on my plan, they decided to register for the same marathon training group and run the race with me. In March 1994, we all crossed the LA Marathon finish line—they both beat me by an hour, but it didn't matter; I could say I'd finished a marathon and had a shiny new medal to prove it!

In time, I expanded my horizons and traveled around the country to experience different marathons, even signing up as a member of the 50 States Marathon Club. My running adventures took me north to Fargo, south to New Orleans, east to Bar Harbor, and west to Maui. And even farther west to New Zealand. Everywhere I went, I'd look around and see that runners came in all shapes and sizes—young, old, tall, short, skinny, fat, and in every imaginable skin color. In the general scheme of things, I was fairly average in the looks and speed department, but I continued to gain self-confidence as I visited new cities, met new people, and tasted amazing local delicacies. I was having the time of my life.

The Accidental Yogist

They say bad things happen for a reason.

It was December 2004, and I had just received notice from my employer that I was going to be laid off. Great way to screw up my Christmas holiday plans, I groaned. But then again, it meant I'd essentially have unlimited vacation time during the holidays. So what to do? I grabbed two male friends and we headed to Yosemite for some winter fun.

It was our first day on the slopes, and I was still trying to break in my brand-new ski boots when it happened. The three of us were getting off the chairlift—two of us went left, the third went right … and because his ski was planted on top of mine, he took my right leg with him as my body veered left. There was a brief moment of panic as I tried to wrestle my ski out from under his. Then boom, I fell.

The anterior cruciate ligament, or ACL, is one of the stabilizing ligaments in the knee. I realized almost immediately that I was in trouble when the cute ski patrol guy helped me to my feet, asked me how I was, and my knee responded by buckling under me. "You've probably torn your ACL," the doctor at the Yosemite clinic later said as he put a splint on my leg. "Go get yourself checked once you get home."

Wanting to get a head start on the recovery process, I made some phone calls. Through pure luck and dropping the right names, I managed to make an appointment with one of the best orthopedic surgeons in LA. He scanned my knee, pronounced it a complete ACL tear, and scheduled surgery for the next month, once the swelling subsided.

Rehab started almost immediately after the effects of the surgical anesthesia wore off. Ice packs, stationary bicycles, weight machines, static exercises, you name it—I wanted to get back to running and checking off the remaining states on my to-do list. The parting words of my orthopod during a post-op visit: No more running marathons for you, my dear; stick to 5Ks instead. He obviously didn't know me, because I traveled to North Dakota soon after and walked another marathon.

The swelling in my post-surgical knee continued to subside, but the flexibility was slow to return. I could only bend my knee until my foot came halfway to my butt. Thoroughly distressed, I researched my options. I'd heard that yoga was good for healing injuries, so I visited my neighborhood yoga studio, registered for the intro special, and gave it a shot. And in time, I was hooked.

The athlete in me loved how my muscles were toning up nicely. The patient in me loved how I was regaining my flexibility. The adventurer in me loved how I could literally drive a mile or two in any direction from home and find yoga studios with a dizzying array of classes and teachers to fit my mood. By then, I'd landed a consulting job, so there was money once again in the piggy bank to fund my newfound yoga obsession. I traveled far and wide, exploring all 4,752 square miles of Los Angeles County. Somewhere along the line, I told a friend about my yoga discoveries and he suggested that I blog about them. Since I was already writing the weekly newsletter for my running group, I thought: Why not? Thus was born my online persona, *The Accidental Yogist*.

I wrote about the many teachers I'd learned from and the many friends I'd made. Yogis and yoginis of all shapes, sizes, colors, and abilities had stories and practices to share that helped enrich my own yoga experience. In time, I was able to give advice on how to talk, dress, and act appropriately for any kind of yoga class, whether it was vinyasa flow, Iyengar, Bikram, Kundalini, Anusara, or power yoga.

I blogged about my journey, my hopes and dreams, my struggles, and my readers offered their experiences and advice. I was part of a worldwide yoga community; we were all in it together. Readers wrote to me and mentioned how much they'd learned from what I had to say. Some people who'd moved to LA from out of town said that they'd found their new home studio through my blog and thanked me for my advice.

I was fortunate to live in Santa Monica, the emerging yoga capital of the Western world. I was a blogging yoga reference manual, and it gave me a sense of satisfaction because I'd worked hard to earn it. I was so embedded in the local yoga culture that the editor-in-chief of the largest and most influential yoga magazine in town reached out to me to join the editorial staff. Accepting her invite was the icing on the cake.

The Changing Face of Yoga

Five years later, after reaching the end of an IT consulting contract and not being able to land a suitable job due to the recession, I attempted to make a living from something, anything, yoga-related. And it was then that I began to see the ugly underbelly of the industry.

Yoga has become the hip new exercise trend. Movie celebrities and rock stars fill the pages of the tabloids as they are photographed leaving yoga classes. I am constantly surrounded by pretty young things in their size 0 lululemon. Thanks to the highly competitive world we live in, yoga has also become a beauty contest and an athletic competition.

It's even gotten to the point where yoga's become all about sex appeal, with yoginis vying to outdo each other in class. Hot yoga classes continue to flood the market, with students parading around in skimpy bra tops and body-hugging shorts. Sometimes I wonder, do they wear skimpy clothes because the yoga's hot, or do they choose to do hot yoga so they can wear the skimpy clothes? Regardless, any woman my age should get her yoga permit revoked for even thinking of trying to compete with them. So I don't even try.

Rather than find enlightenment, the goal of supposed accomplished yogis is to land spots on magazine covers and ad pages. A few years ago I came across an open call for "average-looking" yoginis for a clothing line. Believing I was the epitome of average, I showed up, just to find myself surrounded by room full of yoga sorority girls. Oh, and a very well-known yogini too. I didn't get a callback. I wasn't surprised.

Willing to settle for even a minimal-paying job because the blogging wasn't paying the bills, I applied at three different lululemon stores. Despite having the ideal background—I was a seasoned yogi and runner and had a wealth of experience behind me—I was never called back for a second interview. Was it because I was too short, too old, too pudgy, too ethnic, too wrinkled, not perky enough?

Being able to execute amazing arm balances or backbends help practitioners score high on the yogi popularity scale. Aspiring yoga stars post Facebook photos to elicit likes and comments about how beautiful and sexy they are. After all my years of practice, I still can't manage any pose that makes me look like a balancing human pretzel. People find out that I do yoga and they ask me to demonstrate my skill. Sadly, no one ever seems interested in my mean *savasana*.

But is that really all there is to yoga? Is that what I'm supposed to aspire to be? Is anyone ever complimented for how calm and focused they've become? Or how they can keep from rolling their eyes when surrounded by all the look-at-ME yogis?

Finding My Voice

I'd somehow found myself deep in the midst of an identity crisis. Despite my years immersed in the teachings and practice of yoga, after getting past my dieting days and finally accepting how I looked, how did I manage to end up feeling so inadequate in so many ways?

I wanted to crawl back into obscurity, where it wouldn't matter if I were a middling-looking person with a middling-looking yoga practice. Instead of the long, slim torso that seemed to be de rigueur among the popular yogis, I found myself constantly trying to camouflage my short, thick midsection. And feeling totally frustrated when, despite all my years of taking classes with the best teachers, I still couldn't nail simple arm balances. Then it dawned on me: I'd lived a full and exciting life, traveled the world, raised two well-adjusted kids, and yet here I was, obsessing about the way I looked. Had I lost my mind?

I came to the realization that yoga isn't about *looking* your yoga, it's about *living* your yoga. It isn't about how beautiful your practice is— whether you're a graceful yogini backbending on the sands of a tropical island, or a muscular yogi handstanding at the edge of a rocky mountaintop. What matters most is how you can capture the inner peace and awareness that comes from your practice and share it to make a difference in the world.

Building on my yoga experience, the connections and friendships I'd made along the way, my need to keep discovering new trends and meeting new people, and my ability to speak coherently (at least most of the time), I decided to venture into the world of podcasting. In honor of my not-quite-retired blog, I named my weekly talk show *Yoga Chat with the Accidental Yogist*.

My intent is to provide a forum for others living their yoga: teachers, musicians, filmmakers, authors, health and environmental activists. I always learn something new from them every week; my hope is that my listeners learn something too. Growing an audience can be a popularity contest, but I believe clever conversation trumps brainless blather. This is my chance to stand out, to make a name for myself. And maybe even try to earn a decent living doing it.

So does this mean I'll stop taking yoga classes in public? Not a chance. Whether it be in a yoga studio, on the beach, or at a festival on the top of a mountain, I'll still be that short, middle-aged, average-looking Asian woman in that sea of leggy 20-something aspiring-model blond yoginis. And damned proud of it.

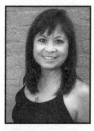

Joni Yung first dipped her toes into the stream of yoga social media when she started her blog, *The Accidental Yogist*. Years later, she took the plunge when she joined *LA Yoga* magazine as a contributing writer, later taking on the role of senior editor. She is now deeply immersed in yoga culture and communication and hosts a weekly podcast, *Yoga Chat with the Accidental Yogist*, featuring interviews with teachers, musicians, healers, and advocates for a cleaner, healthier world. www.yogachatshow.com

Author photo by Sarit Z. Rogers.

PART THREE

Culture and Media

This section looks at the role of mainstream culture and the mass media in shaping our body image. A look at the ways in which a yoga practice can heal body image fractures would not be complete without examining yoga culture. Several contributors examine the "downside" to yoga culture and the ways in which it often replicates the mainstream culture's impossible, and arguably toxic, images of beauty. In the end, this section talks about the ways in which a yoga practice can diminish this cultural noise and argues that culture is what we make—and we can create change that leads to a beauty standard that fits everyone.

Melanie Klein shares her story of alienation and body dissatisfaction, one influenced by family, peers, and media culture. Rooted in resentment and shame, she searched for authenticity, acceptance, and self-value. That path eventually led her to yoga, and the practice weaves with her feminist consciousness and sociological imagination, allowing her to reconnect to her body and combat unhealthy (and distorted) beauty expectations.

Unless he was competing as an athlete, Rolf Gates felt he was a "dirty secret" in a white America. His story includes a tale of recovery from addiction and how meditation and yoga helped build new self-awareness. He also writes about community, culture, and change—ultimately challenging yoga culture to practice what it preaches by moving through its growing pains into the creation of a conscious space for healing.

Next, Nita Rubio talks about the ways in which the female body is objectified in a patriarchal culture, removing ownership and authority from the woman inhabiting that body. She shares her journey home to a place where she is able to create a relationship with the deep wisdom of the female body and move beyond the "male gaze" into a place of reverence and beauty from the inside out.

Seane Corn shares her experiences as yoga cover model and the scrutiny and cultural projections that go with it. As one of the first international yoga sensations, she has aged publicly and been confronted with the rampant ageism that afflicts our culture. Her essay talks about the ways she has combated the trappings of success and continued to evolve into an authentic self more focused on what she does than how she looks—and how that can serve as an example for others.

Chelsea Jackson recounts the pain of feeling like she didn't belong when she began practicing yoga. Despite a desire to walk out of her first class almost immediately, she commits to her practice and learns to accept and embrace her body, see herself as enough, no longer view her body as a burden or inconvenience, and use yoga as a tool of resistance against a culture that often excludes and erases the experiences and voices of members of minority groups.

In an interview with coeditor Melanie Klein, Alanis Morissette relays her experiences of growing into womanhood, a transition that can be challenging enough to any adolescent girl but one made even more challenging when it's done in the body snarking, fat shaming, and scrutinizing light of the entertainment industry. She shares her battle with an eating disorder, her commitment to therapy and personal growth, and how yoga helped guide her integration, connection, and balance.

F*** YER BEAUTY STANDARDS!

Melanie Klein

I felt like shit about my body most of my life.

From age 10 through my late 20s, I resented and battled my body. My body didn't compare to most of the teeny-tiny women in my family. It didn't measure up to the mainstream culture's utterly ridiculous and one-dimensional beauty standards. My body represented weakness, laziness, a lack of self-control, and getting the short end of the stick in the genetics department. Early on, I learned that beauty was a beast, one I had to conquer in order to feel good about myself. And I had to conquer it no matter the costs because, hey, baby, you're worth it.

Roots of Shame

It didn't help that I inherited my stature from the paternal side of my family. I sprung up early and was always the second-tallest girl in class when our teachers would line us up according to height (and I was *always* relieved that the other girl remained on average an inch taller than me all through elementary school). Not only was standing a head above the rest of my classmates awkward, it was like an unwanted spotlight cast upon me at a time when most kids just want to blend in.

My mother and the women on her side of the family were all diminutive with small feet, tiny hands, birdlike shoulders, and itty-bitty waists. They were "delicate flowers" who liked to remind people that they were "petite." I don't think any of them ever weighed more than 110 pounds (and they happily advertised those numbers with fervent regularity), and they all stood under five-foot-two. From the time I'd entered fourth grade, I was referred to as "big-boned," "solid," "big like the other side of her family," and in need of "losing a few pounds." Already measuring five-foot-three and weighing 130 pounds, I was an "Amazon," that poor freak of nature who had inherited the wrong set of genes.

I knew none of these comments were compliments. In fact, most little girls want to secretly flip someone the bird when an annoying aunt or family friend hovers and croons, "My, she's gotten to be such a big girl!" "Big" and "girl" don't go together well in our culture. But I didn't have the confidence or wherewithal to say, "Whoa, whoa, back the hell up. Don't you all know you're talking about my body right in front of me? Don't you know your tones are either derisive or filled with worry about my size? Don't you know this kind of body talk objectifies me and makes me feel like shit?"

Nope, I was too deeply mired in my own shame and guilt about my body. *Why oh why wasn't I born short with a delicate bone structure and "naturally" thin?* I wanted to be short. I wanted to be skinny. I wanted to disappear.

The Body Project

Like too many girls and women, the body was a source of anxiety and shame for the women in my family. The success ("I lost 10 pounds!") and failure ("I gained 10 pounds!") of their "body projects" were a testament of their willpower, a measure of their self-worth, and a barometer of their self-esteem. Like the Plastics in 2004's *Mean Girls* or Carrie, Miranda, and Charlotte from the *Sex and the City* series (Samantha had no problems with her body and she made that clear), the girls and women around me would openly, routinely scrutinize their bodies (and the bodies of others in hushed whispers) as a bonding mechanism and rite of superficial sisterhood.

Body snarking and "fat talk" were a kind of rapport talk, uniting them in the eternal "battle of the bulge." And this kind of rapport talk is not unique to my family. It's a common theme among many girls and women in contemporary culture. While weight is not the only aspect of our body projects (we can lament the size and shape of our breasts, the pimples and wrinkles on our face, and the color and volume of our hair, etc.), it certainly is a focal point.

I remember going to a classmate's birthday party at a Chuck E. Cheese pizza and family entertainment center in the suburban sprawl of the San Fernando Valley. Extra-large silver trays were strewn about, the aftermath of a raucous pizza party for an 11-year-old. Jennifer and I had frosting smeared across our Rainbow Brite T-shirts, and our small, rounded, prepubescent bellies pushed against the waistbands of our wannabe designer jeans, full of pizza and cake. My friend's mom, a former beauty queen who loved diet pills and martinis, pulled each of us in to her bony chest. She squeezed us tight with her thin, bejeweled arms as kids zoomed past us hopped up on birthday cake. With genuine sadness in her voice, she said, "You two will always have to fight your weight." Talk about *heavy*!

You Must Suffer to Be Beautiful

Being a girl seemed daunting. I don't recall hearing the women I grew up with say anything positive about their bodies. There was no sense of wonder or gratitude when it came to their bodies. I never heard them appreciate their health, able-bodiedness, or physical capabilities. What I did hear was a lot of dissatisfaction in the form of griping and nagging.

They openly complained about their flaws and mocked the aesthetic shortcomings of others. From "thunder thighs" to coveted "thigh gaps" to "washboard stomachs" and "wasp waists," every part of the body could be sized up and prove to be a potential hurdle in the pursuit of beauty. And beauty was no easy feat. You had to work for it.

I remember wincing and whimpering one morning as my hair was pulled back too tightly, brushed perfectly smooth, pigtails fashioned and elasticized. "You have to suffer to be beautiful," I was told in response to my protest. It was said tongue-in-cheek, but every joke contains a kernel of truth and I never forgot that statement.

You have to be disciplined. You must exert your willpower. Mind over matter (ignore your hunger! ignore your pain!). You will suffer. But if you succeed, your beauty (read: svelte figure) will not only be a testament to your social worth, but it will bear evidence to your discipline and willpower. Only those of superior mind and body, strength and will, desire and execution will emerge from battle as victors.

And in the numbers game, if you succumbed to a few hundred extra calories, couldn't shake that lingering 10 pounds, or went up a dress size, you didn't just deviate from the cultural beauty norm, you were weak, undisciplined, and bad. Talk about one hundred ways to kill your self-esteem. I felt defeated.

If You Can't Join 'Em, F*** 'Em

Middle school is a cesspool of insecurity, fragile self-esteem, and crises in identity. At least, it was for me. It was as if somebody had cranked up the volume on my body insecurities and shame. What with developing breasts and hips and menses, there were loads of things that could go awry and countless reasons to feel horrible about myself.

I was shy and timid. I didn't want to be seen, and my body language made that evident. I wore baggy tops and my shoulders were so hunched over that I practically turned into myself. Don't get me wrong, I made some attempts to conform, but I wasn't particularly successful. I sprayed Sun-In in my hair to get those sought-after sun-kissed highlights. I began to experiment with mascara, frosted eye shadow, and lip gloss. I started to shave my legs and used skin bleaching cream to lighten my freckles.

The beautiful-equals-thin club was exclusive. I never seemed to be able to get past the velvet rope. At times, I inched close, but I never got in with the beautiful people, the ones seemingly without a care in the world. And because I thought conforming to the beauty norm automatically spelled happiness, I wanted in. I was sick and tired of feeling bad about myself. My lack of willpower and faulty dedication to my body project led to my extra padding—and those extra pounds colored most of my days in less than sunny ways. If I could just lose 10 (or 20) pounds, I'd finally be happy.

Instead of finding the holy grail of weight loss, I found punk rock. It was 1985 and I was 13, full of resentment and repressed anger. My angst was so enormous and stifled that I was bursting at the seams. I immediately resonated with the message, sound, and style of the vagrant, cast-out youth who wanted to turn mainstream society on its head. Unable to join the shiny, happy people I envied, I joined the scuffed-up, angry throng at punk shows and parties across southern California. From Fender's Ballroom in Long Beach and the Country Club in Reseda to backyard parties and abandoned buildings, I'd found a crew of rabble rousers where I thought I belonged. When I couldn't join the ranks of the trendy popular at school, I just gave 'em the middle finger.

Emancipate Yourself from Mental Slavery

Shaving and dying my hair, decades before Gwen Stefani's son, Kingston, was sporting a blue faux-hawk at age 4 without turning too many heads, was liberating and anti-mainstream. But within a couple years, the thrill and satisfaction of aligning with this rowdy counterculture grew stale. It started to feel anything but transgressive.

Ten years ago, as I was finishing my first year as a college professor, a student handed me a film. "Professor Klein, for some reason this movie reminds me of you." I looked down at the copy of *SLC Punk* he'd placed in my hand. I came home and settled in for an incredibly funny and introspective ninety minutes. Set in Salt Lake City in 1986, Stevo and Heroin Bob are one of a few die-hard punks in highly conservative Mormon country. What struck me was that the fictional characters featured in the film were real-life characters that I had met in my own life, albeit a couple thousand miles away. They wore the clothes, or the uniform, my friends and I wore during that same time period. From the music, the behaviors, and the hairstyles down to the black socks, my life and my friends during that period were identical. Not only were we identical to these characters, or tropes, but we were identical to one another. And this was exactly why the punk scene and the "alternative movement" at that time seemed so limiting.

We were drones and slaves to conformity within our own, alternative counterculture. We may have given the finger to the trendies and the jocks that we despised for complying with mainstream expectations, but we set limits on ourselves and the members of our community. We wouldn't *dare* wear something that might be considered uncool by our punk comrades. Two years in, I stepped back and saw that we all looked, sounded, and acted the same. We were just trapped inside another cultural box.

This was the pre–Riot Grrrl era, before an incensed group of sassy young women grabbed their own mics and instruments and challenged the ways the punk community reproduced mainstream sexism and misogyny. I didn't have the language to speak about those issues in 1988, but I did notice that not only were we replicas of one another, the mainstream beauty standards I had so enthusiastically rebuked were present in a group of people I thought had rejected mainstream propaganda. The punk girls who were the most popular and sought after were also the thin, petite girls described as "cute" and "pretty." Aside from their shaved heads or Mohawks, they looked awfully similar to the cheerleaders prancing on the football field and models I saw in ads.

At the end of *SLC Punk*, Stevo's love interest, a rich girl named Brandy, questions him about his blue Mohawk. She asks him if he's trying to make a political statement because, to her, it's much more of a fashion choice devoid of any deeper anarchistic philosophy. She tells him that liberation and freedom aren't authentic when they are dictated by the external world. The film's ending just confirmed what I had felt decades earlier. The punk scene wasn't the answer to the liberation I was seeking.

The F-Word

"It's not you. You're not an isolated case.
It's systematic and it's called patriarchy."—Pat Allen

In 1994, I landed in "Sociology of Women," a class offered as an elective at the local community college I had enrolled in after an extended stint living in Hawaii. When I didn't find the freedom I had longed for in the form of running away by high-tailing it out of Los Angeles with $50 to my name, I flew home on the morning of the Northridge earthquake and went back to school.

Lucky for me, I had enrolled in Pat Allen's class. Pat was a radical 60-something woman who commanded the classroom with a "War is not good for children and other living creatures" medallion swinging from her neck. She lectured with more gusto, authority, and confidence than any woman I had ever encountered. I was utterly smitten and completely enthralled, all the while having my mind blown during each and every class. The world was transformed. My paradigm shifted from one that viewed my body image issues as seemingly personal troubles to understanding them as public issues that were (and are) systemic in nature. In short, my soon-to-be mentor, in all her fierce fabulousness, had ignited my "sociological imagination." And it was distinctly feminist.

My sociological and feminist education included a healthy dose of media literacy, a field of study that was just beginning to blossom at the time. I was offered the ideological tools and skill set to deconstruct mediated images and understand the role of the advertising industry in the creation and manufacture of these endless streams of messages that flood the cultural landscape. This allowed me to examine my tortured relationship with my body in a systematic and structured way, lifting the clouds of shame and guilt that followed my every move.

Maybe there wasn't something wrong with my body. Maybe there was something wrong with the messages the mainstream media culture proliferated, contorted and unrealistic messages that were raking in profits from my insecurity and from the body image issues of girls and women around me. (The mainstream media's targeting of male body image issues didn't begin in earnest until several years later.) The realization that I wasn't the problem was a relief and ultimately liberating. It also left me utterly pissed off.

Welcome to Your Body

Feminism freed my mind. Yoga freed my body. It's one thing to intellectualize self-love and another to embody it. Two years after I stumbled upon feminism's door, I discovered yoga. After years of compulsive and punishing exercise, severe calorie restriction, bouts of binging and purging, and Slim-Fast shakes for breakfast, I stumbled into a challenging but sweet yoga class led by Bryan Kest in an old dance loft in downtown Santa Monica.

The practice and Bryan's rhetoric rocked my mind, body, and spirit. I was shaken to the core. Everything I knew about my body, everything I felt toward my body, and my negative self-talk were about to undergo a seismic shift. For the first time since early childhood, I was about to learn how to be comfortable and radiant in my own skin. For the first time in my life, I was about to learn how to love my body.

I settled in on my mat in a space that would become the rare and sacred space devoid of competition. A space uncluttered by external chatter, removed from the world of advertising, and one that would quiet and soothe my own self-critic. Bryan began that first class by inviting me back into my body, saying, "Welcome to your bodies. Welcome to yoga."

Freedom

I know the yoga industry can be pretty whack a lot of the time, replicating images of beauty replete with all the "-isms" mainstream corporations have been churning out and profiting from for eons. But if you can look past the popularity contests in the yoga scene and the yoga industrial complex that has been manufactured in the last decade and recognize the yoga practice for what it is, you'll see something truly transgressive, if not downright subversive.

I used to think I was giving society a big ol' black-nailpolished middle finger as I would strut down the streets in my Docs and torn fishnets. I thought I was defiant, straight-up revolutionary. Settling onto my mat has been a far more liberating and rebellious act than anything I did or found in that community at the time.

In a world that is increasingly mediated, with ads telling us what we're lacking and how to fill that void and gain self-esteem by using our credit cards, ads that are practically shoved down our throats on every available surface where our eyeballs land, what is more subversive than tuning it all out? My sociological and feminist background had revealed these disturbing trends in the advertising industry and the media at large, but yoga provided the practice as a tool to move inward and craft an inner moral compass on my own terms.

My time on my mat allowed me to tune out external noises, the cacophony of voices competing for my attention and consumer dollars all the while reinforcing an already damaged sense of self. And, simultaneously, my practice soothed the inner voice, ever critical of every detail of my physical self. Uniting breath and movement with intention and focus, I learned how to listen to my body, reconnected with its rhythms and moods, and got to know myself in a way I had not experienced since early childhood.

And with time and consistent practice, my beauty paradigm expanded and shifted. I developed my capacity for patience, empathy, and forgiveness on the mat. These attributes stand in stark contrast to the "no pain, no gain" mentality and value of competition in our culture. As a result of cultivating these qualities and the ability to remain present and be (instead of do through force), my relationship to my body was healed and transformed. My body was no longer an obstacle to be conquered or make over on the road to happiness and love. No, I *embodied* love and I *felt* joy with each practice (and that has never waned in these seventeen years). And there were no numbers on the scale, no amount of retail therapy or consumer consumption, that could or can match that.

My feminist consciousness and my yoga practice provided me the ability to truly shirk repressive and limiting standards of beauty with a big "f*** yer beauty standards."

And mean it.

A portion of this essay was inspired by a longer chapter originally published in Carol Horton and Roseanne Harvey, eds., 21st Century Yoga: Culture, Politics, and Practice *(Chicago: Kleio Books, 2012).*

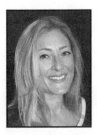

Melanie Klein is a writer, speaker, and professor of sociology and women's studies. She attributes feminism and yoga as the two primary influences in her work. She is committed to communal collaboration, raising consciousness, media literacy, facilitating the healing of distorted body images, and promoting healthy body relationships. Her chapter on yoga, body image, and feminism appears in the anthology, *21st Century Yoga: Culture, Politics, and Practice*, and she is featured in *Conversations with Modern Yogis*. melanieeklein.com

Author photo by Sarit Z. Rogers.

WHAT HAS ALWAYS BEEN

Rolf Gates

Growing up brown in the white America of the sixties and seventies, I was not an expression of my nation's ideals or aspirations, and this point was made clear to me over and over again in every conceivable way. How I looked was wrong, end of story, and that wasn't going to change. The world I grew up in wanted people who looked like me to just go away—unless we were playing a sport. Then we became like a prize racehorse, something thrilling, something to be watched, admired, and possessed. This felt to me to be a far better fate than to live out my existence as America's dirty secret. My body was to be a means to an end. I would spend my youth competing: first as an athlete and later as military officer.

The Buddha taught that we suffer because we believe the impermanent is permanent, the unreliable is reliable, and that things that are not the self are. Nowhere in my experience has that been truer than in the quest to use my body to wrest some measure of respect from a world that would prefer I not exist. By the time I was 14 I had started using drugs and alcohol to manage the traumas and hardships of my daily existence, and by the age of 26 I was a full-blown alcoholic in treatment.

Recovery

My early days in treatment and twelve-step meetings were my first experience of life outside of the culture I was born into. The first thing you notice at a twelve-step meeting is that they declare their ideals and aspirations in a preamble at the beginning of each meeting. The second thing you notice is that everybody appears more than willing to be accountable to the principles expressed in that preamble. As a new person I felt intense shame around my addiction and the mental and physical shape I was in. This did not appear to matter to the members of the twelve-step meetings I attended. Theirs was a culture of recovery and rebirth, and the possibility of my recovery was precious to them. In their world when someone wins, everyone wins.

The consistent expression and adherence to common principles in the meetings I attended created context for me in which I could learn and apply new ways of being in the world. My attitude and outlook were able to change within a culture of rebirth and mutual respect. As I changed, the way I saw the world changed.

Meditation and Yoga

Eventually my program of recovery became a program of self-awareness. One of the first things I noticed after the dust of my active addiction settled was that my body was wracked with a number of different sorts of pain. I had physical injuries from years of using my body to prove something. I had chronic physical tensions from the unresolved emotional trauma of my childhood and my addiction. And my body ached from the constant mental tensions created by the negative habits of mind that filled my days. Twelve-step programs explicitly recommend meditation in their eleventh step. Eighteen months into sobriety, I took them up on it. My first experience of yoga was the practice of seated meditation.

I would sit in a comfy chair, one of my few possessions in early recovery, and set a timer for fifteen or twenty minutes. During that time, I would attempt to count breaths. This remedial form of meditation had an immediate positive effect. The stress I was carrying in my body was cut in half for hours after I meditated. Soon there after, I got wind of yoga poses. The idea of moving in a sacred space, in a sacred way, while incorporating the attention and intention training of meditation sounded really good to me. People would later ask how someone who had lived as I had, spent years knocking people unconscious on playing fields and training with the special forces in the military, came to yoga. If you spent a day in the growing discomfort of my body in my late 20s, you would not need to ask.

Over the years, the combination of yoga poses and seated meditation has more than addressed the mental, emotional, and physical damage inflicted upon my body-mind by a life of trauma. In the beginning, I just felt myself finding more and more ease in my body. I have often said in the classes I teach that the first thing I noticed about yoga was that after practicing the poses, my couch felt better. This physical ease was eventually accompanied by an emotional one. I became less afraid and less angry. With intensive mental training on meditation retreats, I had begun to noticeably increase my overall brain functioning. Empathy for others, imagination, creativity, the ability to think through the consequences of an action, and most importantly the ability to sit with an impulse without reacting have all gathered steam in my life. As I approach 50, I feel as though I am on the cusp of true wisdom and compassion.

Community

When I first came to yoga, I brought my twelve-step culture with me and found a kindred spirit in the yoga community of the mid-nineties. In both the twelve-step world and the yoga world of that time, there was a profound awareness of the number of people finding help within those communities who were healing from sexual trauma as well as other forms of trauma and eating disorders. This awareness fostered a climate of respect for personal space and boundaries that manifested in the possibility of true privacy in one's relationship to their body. In those communities, your body was nobody else's business, and it was understood how painful the use and abuse of your own body could become.

As a young single man going through the trials of my dating years, I cannot remember a single instance in which I commented on a woman's appearance while attending a twelve-step meeting. This sensitivity cut both ways. During those years my self-worth was defined by my ability to live out spiritual principles rather than what I could accomplish with my body or how my body looked.

I attended yoga teacher training about two years before yoga went mainstream in a big way. The summer of 1997 I was seven years sober on my way to a master's program in social work. My attendance at a month-long teacher training program was to be a sober vacation in the Berkshires complete with quiet summer evenings and a lake to swim in. Little did I know that in just two years, everything was about to change.

Looking back, I can see the first rumblings of the mainstreaming of yoga during that summer, but my actual experience holds out real hope for the future of yoga. That summer I was young, strong, and capable, but no one seemed to care. What people commented on was not my appearance; rather, people seemed to like the fact that I lived yoga with all of my heart. The ability to get into this or that posture was almost unnoticed. Most people seemed to feel that if your body could do a pose, great; if it could not, so what? The poses were what you were doing; yoga was how you were being in the pose.

I graduated from that training program with the belief that yoga would make me more at ease in my body so that I could get on with what really mattered. With yoga I could taste life more fully. With yoga I could stand in the poses of my life, the loves, the labors, the works of creation with an ever-increasing ability to balance strength with surrender, wisdom with compassion. That fall I got a new puppy, Max. She ran like the wind through the forests of western Massachusetts; as I walked along behind her, I knew how she felt.

Up to that point, my recovery from my addiction and the culture I had been born into had been a case study in what works. I had been graced to live into the right healing modality at the right time again and again. When I needed to heal from addiction, I found a twelve-step program. When I needed to heal my body and my relationship to it, I found yoga. And when I needed to heal my mind and my relationship to it, I found meditation. In each case the community around the healing practice had created a culture whose principles and actions were aligned with the best interest of the individual. Then a truly huge opportunity happened: yoga got popular.

Sea Change

It is hard to describe what it felt like to have been a part of a very small subculture that had discovered life practices that truly worked and then glimpse the possibility of watching those life practices completely transform a city, an entire class of people, a society, the very world our children would grow up in. In a ten-year period in the United States, the number of yoga practitioners grew from one million to twenty-four million. For better or for worse, I and the other members of the yoga class of 1997 rode that wave.

The process was a little bit like building a frontier town. You use what you have when you have it. Not a lot of thought is given to city planning, and who gets to run things is often a matter of who got there first and who is willing to fight the hardest to run things as opposed to who is best suited for the job. In the case of yoga in the United States, the best method available for quickly adapting to the rapidly growing demand for yoga was individual initiative and entrepreneurship. Most yoga in the United States is taught by a new yoga teacher walking into an empty room and learning to make things happen. It is an incredible story of a relatively few people working largely in isolation creating a societal transformation.

In the hurly-burly of this success story, physical yoga poses were and are being taught skillfully in the United States on a truly massive scale, but the healing context and the intentional community held together by mutually agreed-upon principles were and are not.

My first sense of this and the effect it would have on my relationship to my body showed up in the fall a couple of years after I graduated from my teacher training. I had left graduate school to direct one of the first big yoga studios in the Boston area. I and two other teachers were working hard to meet the demands of a yoga community that seemed to be growing on a weekly basis. We had little time to do anything but teach and found ourselves practicing yoga poses together at work in between classes. That fall I spent a fair amount of time peeking at my peers and comparing myself. Both of my peers were more flexible than I was, and I began to think of myself as kind of average. At some point, getting into "advanced" poses had become both cool and indicative of knowing a lot about yoga. I did not question this shift at the time; I merely noticed that my yoga poses were no longer the sanctuary they had once been.

The "market," our students, really liked the athletic poses, and by providing them our classes grew to unprecedented size. Class size also became an indicator of who was a good teacher and who was not. If you taught huge classes, you were a great teacher. This became a compelling focus for our efforts. Teaching hugely popular classes put the teacher in a position of worldly success that had not been dreamed of just a year or two before. Book deals, clothing lines, and franchises were all in the offing for those who could teach big classes.

The entrepreneurship that drove the growth of yoga also put the student in the position of determining what should be taught. Teaching the poses without the ethical, attitudinal, and meditative aspects of yoga allowed the mainstream culture to co-opt what is now aptly described as the "yoga scene." Within just a few short years, the yoga community as a principle-based healing context ceased to exist.

Creating Culture

This has meant that our society's dis-ease concerning the body, and the many ways this dis-ease is exploited, has had unfettered access to the yoga space. The appearance of success, big classes, small waistlines, and extreme poses have been accepted as the measure of success. In many cases, this has served to amplify an individual's already pained experience with her or his body as they attempt to find health with yoga. In my own experience, the mainstreaming of yoga precipitated a five-year period in which I became a yoga athlete living out the same patterns of proving and striving that I endured as a young person.

With the birth of my first child, the mental and emotional backsliding of my yoga athlete phase was no longer sustainable. My heart yearned for the still space that people can create when they come to-gether around explicitly agreed-upon principles. I began attending med-itation retreats regularly and found myself once again practicing the right modality within the right context. Although it took years, I have been able to undo much of the damage to my relationship to my body, my heart, and my spirit that my time in the "spiritual marketplace" wrought.

Today I feel as though yoga in the United States has undergone nec-essary growing pains and learning experiences—and I along with it. To "roll out" yoga on a large scale, it was attempted to surgically remove the poses from the rest of the practice. It has been an experiment played out on a massive stage and in millions of small ones. I believe what we have discovered with this experiment is that if we are not willing to do the work to create a healing community, the dominant culture fills the vacuum and we cannot realize the potential of our healing practices. Taken as a whole, yoga is the opportunity to heal all of our relationships over time. All that is required is for us to be willing to do the work—all of the work.

A culture is something that we choose for ourselves and for each other. I believe that as we move forward as a community we will prove to have learned from our mistakes and choose wisely. We will create a healing community the likes of which we cannot now even imagine. The spread of yoga as a healing context with mutually agreed-upon principles will spread as rapidly as the spread of yoga as a healing mo-dality.

In my own life, I am also optimistic. I believe I am better for having made the mistakes I made and learned the painful lessons they taught. The most important years of my life are before me, and I have the op-portunity to take what I have learned into being a husband, a father, and a member of the many communities I now call home. I find that if I am willing to act wisely and compassionately toward others, I discover the ability to do the same for myself. It also works in reverse: what I heal in myself, I can heal in the world. My dog Max died in my arms a few years ago, having stood by me through fourteen years of professional yoga teaching. I am now raising my dog Chelsea in the forests of northern California. She runs through the sunlight at peace in her body and in her world, and I am more grateful than ever before to know how she feels.

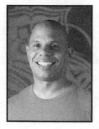

Rolf Gates, author of the acclaimed book on yogic philosophy *Meditations from the Mat: Daily Reflections on the Path of Yoga*, is a leading voice of modern yoga. He conducts vinyasa intensives and 200/500 teacher trainings throughout the United States and abroad. A former social worker and US Army Airborne Ranger who has practiced meditation for the last twenty years, he brings his eclectic background to his practice and teachings. www.rolfgates.com

Author photo by Louis A. Jones.

BEAUTY, VALUE, AND THE FEMININE ROOTS OF YOGA

Nita Rubio

"No," I said.

He asked again whether he could have a drink and hang out with me. My friend and I were on a run to grab more beer from the trunk of our car.

We were on our first summer break after graduation, celebrating with our boyfriends. We felt free and grown-up, yet rebellious. It was a good time held through youth's lens of having all the time in the world at your fingertips. Not a care in the world—except for boys who wanted to drink your beer (and perhaps more) and refused to take no for an answer.

That guy asked us for a beer at least ten times. We knew we were saying no to both giving away our precious cargo and to the subtext of coming along with the beer to "hang out." It was incredibly annoying and invasive. We weren't playing some coy game.

Finally, I said something that I had said hundreds of times before—something that always seemed to work: "We have boyfriends." That was it. It was the kryptonite that loosened their vice grip. As if we had used a wooden stake on a couple of bloodthirsty vampires, they simply shrank back into the night. All I could feel was relief.

My friend and I went back to the party with beers in hand and climbed onto the roof of the vacation house with a dozen or so others to watch the band. I felt distracted and agitated. The feeling did not go away. I sat there for some time with the anxiety running like bees just under the surface of my skin. Something just wasn't right, and I couldn't shake it. Then the answer came in like a lightning bolt: I had to belong to another man for my "no" to be taken seriously—for it to be accepted and honored. My word wasn't enough.

Spontaneous Awakening

Letting someone know I had a boyfriend (sometimes true, sometimes not) was a sentence I had used many times before to get rid of unwelcomed attention. However, I had never once before thought of it in this way. This was like a mallet on my brain. I realized how deeply these men, the culture, and I believed in the men's sovereignty and authority over my own.

This unveiling defined an irreversible change in how I saw myself in the broader cultural context. For the first time, I saw that part of how people perceived me was based on deeply ingrained and taken-for-granted gender stereotypes. Thus began my journey to heal my own relationship to my body and to extricate the ways I had self-objectified, the result of my own enculturation. Being objectified and self-objectifying had created a deep rift between my mind and body.

Coming Home

Several years later I entered a cozy and modest apartment in Silver Lake, California. An altar to a Yoruban goddess named Oshun was in the entryway. Also in the apartment were altars to the Egyptian goddess Sekhmet, the Tibetan goddess Tara, and a few others I didn't know at the time. I had come to study the Tantric Dance of Feminine Power and this was my first class.

At this time, more than fifteen years ago, "Tantra" was not the common word it is today. Hardly anyone knew what Tantric tradition was, including me. I was mainly interested in the other parts of the class title. Dance. Feminine. Power.

My first pilgrimage to this movement modality felt like a sacred oath. I felt like I had finally found an open door to what I knew only in very rare moments in my life: Women Are Magic. No wonder I was nervous.

It turned out in order to access this magic in my body, I would need to confront (and still do) everything in my mind that worked against walking in the world liberated from all my own self-deceit and self-hatred. I would need to stand in my own inner power in a world that did not want me to be liberated from these things.

From the Inside Out

This movement modality was originated and developed by my teacher, Vajra Ma. It is a practice of the subtle body. There are no techniques, dance steps to learn, or mirror to watch yourself in. The movement must come from deep inner feeling.

The subtle energy expresses itself and shapes the body into gestures and full body mudras (postures that seal the energy in a certain configuration within the body). Through my continued education in the traditional lineages of Tantra, I learned that it is precisely this type of meditation and inner communication that the ancient yoginis used to develop the yoga *asana* practice.

I was taught that *asana* practice was originally used as medicine. The medicine was to be used in certain ways, during certain times in a female practitioner's life, and in tune with the moon, to which we are inextricably linked. I loved learning about the relationship between the wisdom of the female body and the wisdom of the cosmos—that this relationship to the deep wisdom within the female body and the deep wisdom of the movement of the cosmos were not separate things and that a woman can find her place among the earth and the stars in an incredibly real and nonconceptual way.

The most important thing about this practice is that it was fluid and dynamic. The internal energies, the menstrual blood that we are tuned to in our cycles, and nature are all fluid. It is movement that is the hallmark of the feminine roots of yoga. As you learn to move with the internal energies, you learn how to move with life's flow. Beauty emanates from here because it is deeply rooted from within.

Beauty—but Not Like You'd Think

Reverence of beauty is not a new thing. Beauty has been exalted for thousands of years, according to the surrounding cultural and political mechanisms that define a society's norms and moral values. This has also crept into current spiritual pursuits. Those with the looks, money, confidence, and right affirmations will secure their place and hold court in the popular club. As they do, they push the "are we good enough" buttons of the rest of us who desire to be included.

In great traditions such as yoga and Tantra today, the current barometers of being rich, white, popular, and thin have infiltrated the field, further perpetuating patriarchal paradigms that being beautiful, successful, and, yes, a consumer gives you value and worth as a human being. This is a long way from the roots of yoga and Tantra. The further away from the roots we get, the easier it is to forget what truly informs our value not only as spiritual practitioners but as human beings.

Interestingly enough, beauty is at the root of our source as human beings. It is at the root of yoga and Tantra—and it is a great teaching. But today its corpse lies in the shadow of spiritual branding and all externally based systems of value.

In the Tantric cosmology, we all come from beauty. This beauty is not one based on a standardized list of perfection. Nor does it reference an ideal. This beauty is based on feeling. Beauty is an experience. Feeling is the precise wisdom that beauty holds. When we encounter beauty, we come out of the stream of thought and are completely in the moment. Think of the times you have gazed upon a magnificent sunset. You don't say such things as "Oh, that was a magnificent sunset, but the one I saw back in 1982 was much better." We don't compare this beauty. Its beauty comes from resting in its inherent nature.

As a teacher of the Tantric Dance of Feminine Power, I have seen hundreds of women experience their own beauty in this way. Their experience comes from a radical acceptance and even a reverence of the intelligence in their own bodies. They have become something more than a list of bullet points of perfection. By being completely immersed in the naturalness of who they are and how they feel, they liberate themselves from the stream of critical thought and encounter the source of their own beauty within. And it has energy and movement! This is a huge contrast to a lethargic two-dimensional pouty image in a magazine.

The Tantric Dance of Feminine Power was the ignition for my passion that arose for deep feminine beauty and authentic power. I found these roots of the ancient yoginis every time I entered the dance. All of the profoundly simple guidelines of the practice ensured that I was continually drawing on my inner wisdom, meaning I had to feel all the deep internal movements of my body. The more I did this, the more awareness developed of the immensity of territory within myself, terrain that had nothing to do with how I measured up against any model of frozen perfection. There were experiences within my body that affirmed my value again and again. The criteria of value were based upon the simple fact that my body housed a cosmology of wisdom. This wisdom was in harmony with my mind and with an intelligence that infuses all beings and things with a vibrational dance that tells us we have more in common than our limited sufferings of the "I."

The Community of Women

It was not merely my own inner experience that produced these transformations. My journey was deeply guided by and tied to the other women's journeys in the classes.

Comparison and competition between women is a pervasive disease. I cannot recall a time before my awakening that summer break when I was encouraged to feel what another woman was feeling. I cannot remember a time when I had been in contact with women who felt themselves from the inside out and did not act out their beauty hand-in-hand with some kind of neurosis (such as compulsive shopping or disordered eating). I cannot remember a time when I saw real images of women's pleasure or saw women experiencing their own erotic connection to themselves and life at large.

No, all the women I knew, including myself, were trying to fit into the perfected form of happiness that was based on an externally identified sexuality, as an object of desire. The act of "witnessing" (instead of watching) the other dancers, an important part of the Tantric Dance of Feminine Power, was and continues to be a profound experience for both myself and the many students I have had throughout the years. I call it "letting go of the pretty." This is code for letting go of all the ways women view themselves from the outside in and the knee-jerk reaction to being "perfect" as dictated by the dominant culture.

Women in my classes are encouraged to allow asymmetrical movement, facial expressions that distort the face (I mean, come on, do we really think a woman's face in deep pleasure looks like the ones we see in the movies?), and movements that "don't seem to make sense." The outcome is deep and esoteric. Women begin to tap into a wildness that has nothing to do with the "girls gone wild" fast food and violent sexuality we've been spoon-fed by media conglomerates.

Our wild nature does not lie in the gestures created by a culture that wants to turn women into the ultimate consumers by constantly telling them they are not thin enough, sexy enough, or desirable enough. Our wild nature lies in the joyful experience of being a creature of nature— and remembering that we are nature. Our wild nature lies in the recognition that we are unowned, alive, and tremoring with the pulsations of life—not some emulation of a perfected life with a frozen grin. We are blood and bone, fire and grit, saliva and sweat, encased around a pearl of such exquisite softness that it puts to shame those who look for the holy grail elsewhere.

When freed from the patriarchal gaze upon our bodies and experiences, women tap into a self-reference and freedom that are innate and natural. One of my most memorable moments is when a longtime student quietly declared that she had never experienced herself as her own guide before.

Betraying Myself

All this existed in that first class I attended years ago. I witnessed a woman in her dance. She began in deep stillness, deeply connected to her womb (the seat of Goddess in the Tantric tradition), and, oh, I felt her! After a brief minute she had gone so deeply internal that I could not recognize her face anymore. She was moving and shape-shifting. The twitches in her face revealed that it was this internally sourced path of ecstasy that shaped all of her gestures—gestures that I recognized to be the root of the yoga *asanas* as we know them today.

She was transmitting power, and I received healing from that power. It was an overflow from her deeply felt experience into the room and into all of us who witnessed. I was astounded. Little did I know this would begin a deep healing and dissolving of all the ways I viewed myself and other women through the lens of patriarchal gender norms and stereotypes.

Why did this particular woman shock my system and awaken this process within me? She was awake and alive. She was intoxicated with the power and feeling of her own body. It had nothing to do with me, yet it had everything to do with me. It was then and there that something wilder, more primal, and more courageous beckoned me. It was this transmission of power that opened the door for the shadow of my own self-betrayal to emerge and be offered up at the altar of Woman for healing.

For years I had been betraying myself by constantly criticizing my belly, hair, skin, and more. Betrayal was etched into my bones every time I looked in the mirror and deemed I wasn't worthy of everything that perfection said it would grant me. Interestingly, every time I looked in the mirror it was my belly I focused most of my critique on. I say this is interesting as now, through Tantric practice, I know that the belly, womb, and vagina are considered potent places of power for women. These places of power had received my most intense judgments. I was betraying myself by shutting down deep belly feeling and trading it for trying to make myself smaller both literally and figuratively. I cannot even remember how young I was when this started. It seems to have always been there, which is a frightening thought.

Like a fish that doesn't recognize it is swimming in water, it's only in hindsight that I realize the profundity of what was missing in my life, the circle of women who could reflect my own experience of my body, spirit, and mind. I'd certainly never seen "real" female bodies. I had been trained, through the prolific repetition of images of Photoshopped "perfection" in media and celebrity culture, to not see or to reject real live women with an immediacy and efficiency that is alarming.

My value system was entirely based upon this process of weeding out those who didn't measure up to the cultural standard of beauty. If I wasn't doing that, I was spending my time comparing myself to those who were left, trying to see where I fit—vying for space. Using the criteria of digitally altered body "perfection" led me to further disconnect from my body and to create relationships based upon fragile and vulnerable ground. After all, how could the ground for relationship be stable when it's based upon seeking external approval and admiration? That is a breeding ground for endless pain.

Coming into Wholeness

My journey with body image and healing is one of Desire and Union. It was the embracing of the female reverent lineages of traditional living Tantric streams that provided a container and a context for actually becoming an embodied, rather than disembodied, woman.

Interestingly, it wasn't the frozen, symmetrical, balanced, and well-known yoga *asanas* that helped to heal my relationship to my body. It was specifically the shamanistic and feminine roots of yoga, the inspiration of female practitioners illuminated by authors Vicki Noble and Miranda Shaw, as well as my fortunate opportunity to sit with teachers such as Vajra Ma and Parvathi Nanda Nath who live this fluid yoga of beauty and power.

Asana is translated as seat. In the Tantric tradition, this seat is a seat of power. It is to be able to rest in the natural ground of one's being and find the unlimited source of life's flow, grounded through being in your body. This life flow is called Shakti, which is power, energy, and it is moving. Practiced in this way, each *asana* gives you the chance to come home to your body.

Unfortunately, the *asanas* as we have come to know them have become distanced from the primordial feminine energy that is Shakti. She is hardly referenced, and what has entered in her absence is rigidity and sterilization of an originally ecstatic practice of the female yoginis and shamans.

Do I still practice the *asanas* that are prevalent in the West? I do. But what comes with me to the mat now is my already intact sense of wholeness and value based upon being in a lineage of women who have found sovereignty within themselves. I bring my womb and breasts to the mat. I bring the blood mysteries within myself. I bring my love for Goddess as She has been known since the beginning of time. I bring the sense of resting in myself and resting in each *asana* as the seat of power.

I see with a discerning eye how the images of women, even in yoga, continue to push the "good enough" button. Does this button continue to get pushed in myself? Yes, oh, yes. It's a button thousands of years in the making. It's a beast. But I love the beast too. This is also Goddess. I bring my devotion to Her to the mat as well. She was there in the roots of yoga. I see Her now showing up for women in my classes, giving them choices to enter their "imperfections" and their own "beasts" and say, "This is me, also."

Yoga is a rich experience for me now. I taste it all, digest it through my own ecstatic experience, and allow my body to be a vehicle of intelligence. To become inner-referenced rather than externally defined is one of the greatest joys I have known.

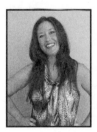

Nita Rubio (Nisha Bhairavi) is a yogini in the Kaula Shakta Tantric tradition. She is a master teacher of the subtle body movement modality, The Tantric Dance of Feminine Power®. Embodiment, traditional Tantric lineage practice, feminism, and ritual intersect in Nita's offerings. Joyfully teaching for over seventeen years, it is her great passion to weave these traditions without diluting their potency both in the classroom and personally into a continuous stream of Feminine Wisdom in Action. www.embodyshakti.com

Author photo by John Colao.

POWER, PRIVILEGE, AND THE BEAUTY MYTH

Seane Corn

The truth is, growing up I never really had a negative body image issue. Of course, like every other young girl, I looked at all the magazines and compared myself to the models and knew I fell way short of the stunningly beautiful women I'd see. I wished I had their long legs or straight, smooth, blond hair or perfectly symmetrical face completely devoid of ethnicity.

At various times I might have looked at my body and face and said, "I should probably do something about that." "That" being perceived as a "flaw" or a "problem." But, more often than not, I couldn't be bothered, and I didn't obsess. The media images did not impact my self-esteem the way they seemed to for many of my friends, especially for those of color or who weren't stick skinny. I was naturally thin and had enough qualities in my face and body to include me in a part of that standard of beauty that allowed me many seen and unseen privileges, and, as a result, supported me to feel fairly self-confident and at ease in my youth.

My friends, on the other hand, had little or no examples of people who looked like them represented in these magazines. I could see it made them feel inadequate and unrecognized, and for a couple of them, even enforced some deeper feelings of worthlessness that I didn't understand at that time. Many of my friends developed eating disorders, starving themselves to lose weight. Some would straighten their hair, get nose jobs, and even lighten their skin. Pictures of the models they aspired to look like hung on their walls, and they'd spend countless hours trying to change who they were to replicate the images of these women, even though they were often of a different race or impossible body type.

Today, I am well aware of how these conventional beauty standards are specifically designed to objectify, disempower, and purposely make us feel like we need to change into something "better"—meaning different than who we already are. These standards are racist, ageist, fat shaming, and rarely, if ever, acknowledge those with disabilities. They are used to manipulate us in many ways, including separating us from our money—so we can buy the necessary products to "help" us reach our beauty goals—and each other, perpetuating the historical hierarchy of power that has alienated and oppressed so many.

There is a projected ideal of youth and beauty that exists, and we have been seduced and manipulated to believe that if we fit into that ideal we will be happier, healthier, and more adored, desired, and perhaps even loved.

I'm also well aware of how, as a featured yoga model in health and wellness magazines, I've participated in this projection and perpetuated the homogenization of the standard of beauty as a result.

Positive Attention?

My yoga career popped on a local level in 1995, and by 1997, I was teaching nationally. The momentum was like a tsunami, and I knew it wasn't because I was the most brilliant yoga teacher there was. Far from it. I was a lot of things, but I wasn't a good teacher yet. In fact, I was young, insecure, and inexperienced. I also began to get a lot of media attention, including being on *The Today Show* and shooting covers and editorials for yoga magazines within months of completing my first teacher's training. My fast-tracked success was about timing, luck, and to be very frank, the fact I happened to fit into a certain physical mold, a specific look that people seemed attracted to: I was thin, flexible, strong, pretty, and white. I fit into a mainstream ideal that could be marketed and used to help commercialize yoga.

Although I was excited by the opportunities I was getting and thrilled to see myself in the pages of magazines, I also knew I was perpetuating an unrealistic perception of health and wellness based on my personal genetics. Over the years, I continued to see women of my race and body type represented in print almost exclusively. It saddened me to see the way that the yoga community, including myself, was contributing to the ongoing and disempowering myths of beauty that diminish and dismiss the majority of women and girls who don't fit that limited and narrow ideal.

As yoga became more popular, and more commercial, I would often ask myself that if an aspect of yoga is about the interdependency, relationship, and unification of *all* beings, then why wasn't that diversity represented in the marketing? Where were the examples of people of color? The disabled? The heavyset? The old? If yoga teaches us to let go of the ego and our attachment to outward identification, and to look inward for value, why was an unrealistic physical ideal the face of American yoga? This creates separation and, intentionally or not, reflects an image of yoga that is elitist, exclusionary, skinny, and very, very white.

As the attention on me increased and I became even more visible, I had one of those moments of awareness—ah, so this is how this is going to be for me ... I'm going to get opportunities and be awarded privileges that many other teachers, even more talented teachers than myself, won't receive, and more often than not it's going to be because of how I look. This awareness was humbling, especially because I knew I had a lot more to offer than my image. I also knew that all the validation and attention I was receiving was a seductive and incredibly attractive trap, and I gave a lot of thought to how I was going to navigate it.

I had a couple choices. I could personalize it and make the attention all about me and endlessly feed my ego with all the supposed love and appreciation I was getting. Or I could truly work hard on developing a strong sense of self and earn the attention I got in a way that was authentic and honoring of all yoga practitioners. This meant that I would have to keep evolving in my own personal process, take responsibility for both my light and my shadow, and work toward becoming an articulate, generous, and well-informed teacher.

In time, I also realized that I could use the way I've benefitted from my privileges and utilize my public platform responsibly by redirecting the attention onto things that are way more vital and important, using my influence to inspire personal growth and even perhaps global action. This was the only way I could make sense of what was happening to me. I wasn't a model, I wasn't invested in my popularity, and I wasn't attached to yoga as a career. I was a deeply committed and passionate student and realized that I suddenly had some interesting karma to work through. I wanted to be as conscious in the process as possible. This included looking at my success.

I understood early on that success ebbs and flows, often at the whim of trends and public opinion. I didn't want my success to define me and live my life attached to maintaining it. In the same way, I didn't want my beauty or youth to determine my self-worth. I was given a gift and wanted to use the platform and opportunities I was given purposely and well. I wanted to commit to myself in my personal practice and teaching to inspiring empowerment, healing, and—what has become the dedication of my life—being of service.

Focus on the Body

During this early period in my career, what I wasn't prepared for was the projections and the amount of attention and scrutiny my actual body got and my reaction to it. I became very self-conscious and entirely too aware that parts of me weren't "perfect." I would fret the week before a shoot, restricting my food intake and increasing my time on the mat, for no other reason than to help tone my muscles a bit more. I was aware that the opinions about my body would only grow as I continued to be photographed and consumed by the public, and it scared me. I felt the pressure and insecurity that many women feel—that I didn't stack up, wasn't pretty enough, wasn't thin enough, wasn't perfect. I felt inadequate.

So I sat with the feelings that came up. Breathed into them. Investigating my relationship to body image became a part of my yoga and healing at that time, and I did a lot of work on myself to remember what was truly important (most certainly not the size of my ass) and what I was committed to standing for (self-acceptance). I decided that if being publicly visible and a "cover girl" were going to be a part of my journey, then I needed to contribute in a positive way to how women were perceived… starting with myself.

One of the things I request when asked to pose for a magazine is that I cannot be Photoshopped without consent. This was, and remains still, an issue for me, as this is a process that sets up the unrealistic ideals that we as a culture often desire and can never realize because it's a lie. Photoshopping and good lighting create an image that does not exist in reality. The women you see in the magazines do not look that way in life. Recently I was Photoshopped on the cover of a magazine to the point where I look like a 12-year-old girl. My skin was flawless, my eyes were brightened, and the lines around my mouth were nonexistent.

I can understand getting rid of a zit in the middle of my forehead or smoothing out the wrinkles in the outfit I'm wearing, but I'm not comfortable when I am altered to look other than the way I am. I've been Photoshopped in the past where the companies I've worked for have given me larger breasts, narrowed my waist, taken down my thighs, flattened my belly, elongated my neck, and/or thinned out my upper arms. Even though I'm drawn to the illusion of flawlessness they give me, I know it's not the truth of who I am and how I look. They have also tried to fill in the very obvious scar that runs through my right eyebrow—a scar that in my youth was a source of discomfort and that I used to fill in with makeup so that my face would be "normal." At 18 I decided to reclaim this tiny imperfection as a unique part of who I am and vowed never to cover it again.

I've had to call these companies and tell them that I can't be represented in a way that is not truthful. It's not what I stand for. First of all, while I may sort of like those breasts, they're not mine and it's not an authentic representation of who I am. It is now in my contracts that I have final approval of all photos that get released. In the case of the recent cover photo where I'm practically unrecognizable, I did not approve that photo and it should not have been published as it was. No one was more surprised than me when I saw it on the newsstand, and I felt sad to see my face devoid of experience, character, and age. Photoshopping is an ongoing issue that continues to marginalize women and perpetuate the myths and idealization of standardized beauty. The older I get, the more I know Photoshopping is going to increasingly be an issue and something that I will continue to fight against.

Body Image and Aging

As a 47-year-old woman I am working hard not to allow these standards of beauty interpret how I approach aging and the way I feel about my body or myself. I intend to embrace aging in a way that is celebratory and unapologetic, which are things that I feel strongly compelled to stand for in my life. I do feel the push-back from society that says aging is bad, scary, undesirable, etc., but I don't want to participate in this level of limited and fear-based thinking and minimize my experience of life as a result.

Many people don't believe that I'm comfortable in the aging process (including the client who offered me Botox and Restylane as my 40th birthday present), and this is because there's such an ingrained stigma associated with aging in women that has become the norm. I'm fully aware that at a certain age, women simply disappear—we become invisible. As our body changes, we don't get the same kind of attention, adoration, reverence, or respect. We become marginalized.

In the almost twenty years that I have been teaching, I have been on twenty-four covers and in countless editorials. I will have two more covers coming out next year. I think it is wonderful that I'm pushing 50 years old and still getting asked to be on the cover of magazines that promote health. I celebrate this. What I don't want is to be portrayed as a "beautiful" 47-year-old because I'm made to look like I'm in my 20s; this diminishes the authentic image of a healthy 47-year-old that I have an opportunity to be a role mode of.

As a leader within the yoga community and a public figure, I am well aware that there is a certain amount of projection and even expectation to look and be a certain way physically, spiritually, and ethically. Although conscious of it, I choose not to be defined by it or live my life fitting into someone else's projection of how I should look, behave, or be. I have had experiences where people meet me and tell me that I am shorter than they thought I would be, or I am not as thin as they expected, telling me that I'm "so much juicier" than my pictures. They will say in whispered tones, "I can't believe you're almost 50!" as if it's something I'm keeping a secret. I've even been told that I don't look Jewish (my religious heritage). What does a Jew even look like? Is it good that I don't? Bad? These comments are not overtly negative, but there are unconscious undercurrents that perpetuate ideals and stereotypes that I often feel the pressure to fit into. An ideal that, ironically, I perpetuated myself!

I never want to apologize for the natural process of aging or shame myself for the inevitable changes in my body that will continue to come. As I age, I see my father in my face in a way I never saw before. I welcome this. I want to own my changes, celebrate them, and honor them. I hope to inspire other women to embrace their unique beauty and allow for their own organic changes to happen gracefully. I also have no interest in trying to re-create the body of my youth as I age publicly. If I did try to fit those conventions, and conform to those ideals, I would miss the incredible experiences that aging brings—including perhaps deep self-acceptance, heart-embracing empathy, and fierce wisdom.

I earned this age. I'm fortunate to still be here in this body, and I hope to have many, many more years upon this earth to grow, expand, and become more self-realized. If this means that my hair may thin, my jowls soften, my breasts sag, and my waist expand, so be it. It is just this cycle of life, birth to death, that yoga teaches us to not become attached to and then ultimately transcend. It is sad that we become marginalized just at the same time we become our most fabulous!

Inside Out

So although I recognize that I am in a culture, and in a business, where there is a lot of body idealism with ongoing pressure to fit into that ideal, I will continue to work diligently not to buy into a collective projection of what beauty is as manufactured by a team of marketers who are invested in keeping us insecure. For me, beauty is a process of being that radiates from the inside out and is in direct relationship with our capacity for love. I'm glad that I am one representation of beauty, but beauty isn't, nor will it ever be, limited to color, size, gender, age, ability, or culture. Beauty is who we are in relationship to spirit, not our outward appearance as determined by society.

I apologize for the ways I perpetuated the myth that beauty is a certain shape, size, and color, but I'm glad to now be in a position where I can raise awareness about it. I am hopeful that as we in the yoga community (and the world) grow, we can recognize the ways we have been complicit and continue to acknowledge the broad and endless range that beauty truly is, and celebrate its ever-evolving and differentiated face, especially in our magazines and marketing. Yoga brings us into a deeper relationship with Self, but this can never be obtained if we continue to marginalize people based on their appearance. We need to evolve the standards of beauty to be more inclusive and representative of the myriad shapes, size, colors, genders, and ages that exist. We need to model back to the world the ways in which we refuse to contribute to historical oppression within marketing that keeps people repressed, insecure, and separated.

May we recognize the opportunities we have to shift perception as a collective and work diligently to create a global standard of beauty that celebrates *all* beings as beautiful. May we commit to honoring each precious and unique soul as valued, honored, and loved ... for exactly who we are.

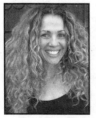 **Seane Corn** is an internationally renowned vinyasa flow yoga teacher and spiritual activist, who focuses her teachings on self-empowerment, self-actualization, purpose, and inspired service. Since 2007, she has been training leaders of activism through her cofounded organization Off the Mat, Into the World. Seane is also cofounder of a groundbreaking fund and awareness effort across the yoga world called the Seva Challenge Humanitarian Tour, which has col-

lectively raised over $3.5 million since 2007 for international communities in need. Her five self-authored DVDs and CD set are available through Gaiam, *Yoga Journal*, and Sounds True. www.seanecorn.com

Author photo courtesy of the author.

TOO MUCH AND NOT ENOUGH

Chelsea Jackson

The moment I walked into that hot-ass room I was pissed. Staring at the reflection of my 200-pound, five-foot-five frame while looking around at the white and svelte sweaty bodies, I seriously thought of quietly rolling up my mat and tiptoeing to the nearest exit. Laughing in their designer sports bras as they bounced to their mats, no one really said a word to me, but then again I didn't really try making eye contact with anyone either. *What am I doing here?* I thought to myself. I didn't even want to look at my reflection for too long because it made me panic even more. My own eyes staring back at me, I recognized decades of pain and frustration that had been ignored and dismissed. There I was in this ridiculously hot room, in an oversized T-shirt that I hoped was big enough to cover the layers of cellulite I had grown to be ashamed of.

Truth is, I wanted to strip down to my sports bra underneath too, but in my mind I was too big and too brown in this endless sea of fit and white female bodies. I was unsure of how people would look at me; however, one thing was clear, I no longer needed the abusive reminders from my gymnastics teacher and middle-school cheerleading coach telling me I was not good enough. I'd learned the art of body shaming just fine on my own.

You're too big, I thought. *You will pass out for sure if you go through with this.* But instead of running, I decided to stay. I decided to confront myself with myself and look at my image staring back at me. My full hips, my stretch marks, my straightened hair that was slowly transforming into an Afro right before my eyes were all things I realized I resented in that moment. My brown body was an inconvenience for me in certain places.

By the time I took my first yoga class, my body had already endured two decades of ridicule for being too big, too curvy, or just not the right body type for particular spaces that little girls often dream of fitting into. Why would yoga be any different? After all, I only saw maybe one or two women of color on the cover of a particular yoga publication I obsessed over before building the nerve to attend that first class. In addition to that, I never had the pleasure of seeing someone who actually had curves like mine engage in something that emphasized the body as much as yoga. Moments before the instructor walked in, flashbacks from my childhood and the experiences that contributed to my relationship with my body convinced me that my presence in this space was a mistake. Perhaps I should just quit before I embarrassed myself any more than already had.

Too Much and Not Enough

It wasn't that I thought I would become a professional gymnast or anything, but it was something about the way she said it that made me think it could never be an option. Constant remarks by my gymnastics coach such as "Tuck in your butt, Chelsea" made me feel I had failed. Failed by no effort on my part other than walking in a black girl's body. Through my gymnastic coach's verbal reminders, and occasional taps on the backside, I was encouraged to diminish my physical presence in order to look like a gymnast. I developed a relationship with my body by the age of 6 that allowed others to define the borders surrounding my body. What I could do, what I shouldn't ever try doing, and the rules for where my body was appropriate were established.

In addition to the curves attached to my strong, adolescent, a female body, brown skin, and kinky hair further complicated the ways in which

I saw myself fitting in as a gymnast. Despite my parents' countless efforts to surround me with dozens of black Cabbage Patch dolls, Africa Barbie, and even a black version of that creepy talking Cricket doll, my lived experiences at Saturday morning gymnastics sent the message that I did not belong in certain worlds. Worlds that welcomed some and shamed others impacted me more than I could ever comprehend in the first grade. I practiced how to diminish my presence in order to blend in or make others feel comfortable despite how damaging it was to my physical body and psyche. Whether it was by shrinking my height and collapsing my shoulders in my fifth-grade class picture to appear as petite as most of the other girls in my class, or by learning how to wear two sports bras to minimize the size of my breasts, I cultivated the skill of lessening myself in order to fit in.

Eventually, I pleaded with my mother to discontinue my participation in gymnastics without fully understanding or being able to articulate why it was I lost interest in the first place. Later, I attended tryouts for my school district's Pee Wee Cheerleading team, and between the ages of 8 and 18, I participated in national cheerleading competitions and became the captain of cheerleading squads. My ability to tumble and memorize cheers made my presence on cheerleading squads unquestionable; however, once I entered high school I was met with some of the unresolved feelings I had about my body as a 6-year-old gymnast. As I moved through middle school, I had noticed a stronger emphasis placed on the physical appearance of cheerleaders by peers and coaches. "Weighing in" at the end of cheerleading practice and having our measurements announced in front of the squad was a regular routine and became a source of anxiety for me each week.

"One of you actually weighs 165 pounds; you all are getting too fat to be cheerleaders!" I vividly recall my coach announcing during one of the weigh-ins. Mortified that I was the cheerleader who weighed 165 pounds, I immediately retreated to my 6-year-old self who wanted to abandon a space that rejected who I was and how I looked. Although I had been able to perform the role of a cheerleader successfully since I was a child, I was beginning to notice the messages being sent during my teenage years telling me that my body no longer belonged in this space either. Unlike my experience as a young gymnast, I stayed. By the end of my junior year I attempted to gain control over my body by depriving myself of what entered my body and seeing how quickly I could make it exit. The fear of hearing my weight called as the largest girl on the squad overtook my body, and during a short period of time I learned the art of both starving myself and forcing food out of my body in order to avoid this rejection.

I was not the only cheerleader on my squad concerned about weight and size; some girls began smoking cigarettes once they realized the habit suppressed their appetite. Some learned how to eat small portions of food really slowly, while others mastered the art of skipping meals without their families noticing. What made these practices most disturbing and at the same time sustainable was the fact that so many of us were practicing them together. On one occasion when I thought I was alone in the school bathroom during a team pizza party, a fellow squad member listened in the stall next to me as I attempted to stick my finger down my throat in order to release the multiple slices of pizza I just devoured. I feared that she would tell friends or our coach; instead, she informed me that I wasn't doing it correctly and showed me the most efficient way to vomit.

My eating disorder did not last very long, but it did exist. It existed in a way that not only damaged me physically, but also influenced the ways in which I would later respond to stress throughout adulthood. On the one hand, the stress of maintaining an "acceptable" body type catapulted me into a false sense of control that was extremely restrictive in terms of what I ate and how much I ate. On the other hand, stress also created a response that disregarded healthy boundaries, causing me to overeat and feel guilty about my decision later. This dance between too much and not enough not only showed up in my relationship with my body and food, but it also left me deeply disconnected from the core of who I was and the root of why I responded in this way.

Throughout college and early adulthood, stress would show up in various ways. From seemingly small and fleeting moments such as homesickness and heartbreaks to extremely traumatic times including the murder of my best friend, my responses to stress were consistent.

Depending on the type of response my stress triggered, I would go back and forth between the "not enough" and "too much" behavior. Unable to hide the consequences of these patterns, stress could always be detected by my body becoming extremely thin or significantly fuller. This volatile and damaging relationship endured for the early part of my adult life, leaving me with huge fluctuations in my weight, high cholesterol, and brief periods of depression. By the second semester of my freshman year in college, I was overwhelmed by my size and became discouraged when I couldn't keep up with my mother during our walks in the park. I was disconnecting from myself and wanted desperately to feel whole again. I wasn't really sure of how to go about that; however, I did know that I wanted to finally feel confident and secure in my body regardless of the space I was in. It wasn't until four years later that I would walk into my first yoga class.

In Search of Wholeness

My love for yoga was not "at first sight." I wasn't a fan of yoga on the first try and reluctantly tried it a second time. Honestly, I was not sure if it was something for me because I didn't see a lot of *average*, not to mention overweight, folks like me showcased in advertisements, magazines, or the few instructional videos I previewed before attending my first class. I tried yoga because I was out of options. I was out of ways to figure out how to resist patterns that caused so much suffering, not just in my body, but throughout my life. I wanted to move beyond just losing weight, and I knew the moment I looked into my eyes in that hot room, yoga would kick my ass by forcing me to ask the question—why? Why is it so difficult to look at myself? Why am I so resistant to this? The internal questions during class wouldn't stop and I couldn't turn my mind off.

"Remember to breathe in slowly while looking into your eyes," whispered the instructor, slowly weaving in and out of the three rows.

During mid-inhale I began to ask myself why there were no other black women, or simply nonwhite people, in this class with me? Then I began to think that it is probably counterintuitive to ask questions that have the potential to piss me off in the middle of a yoga class.

"Soften your gaze on the exhale," the instructor mentioned while pausing near my mat. I'm convinced she heard the conversation going on in my head.

"How can I soften when all of these feelings are coming up?" I thought as I continued my practice. Gradually, my fear turned into anger as I thought more about the answers to my questions. In that moment my practice became not only about the image in front of me, but the other images similar to mine that were absent from the room and might be asking some of the same questions I had. Answers to my 6-year-old self who wanted to know why her backside was not *appropriate* and made her coach feel so uncomfortable. I wanted to know why as a young adult, I still felt like the same teenage girl who was terrified of being marginalized because of her size.

Although a whirlwind of emotions moved through my body and mind during that 90-minute class, I was also able to tap into a place I had never traveled before. It was a place filled with both fear and courage. It was a place where I felt both empty and full. It was a place where not enough and too much existed for me, but this time I wasn't afraid of them. It was a place that finally began to pull the curtain back on what had been the root of my pain for so many years: my invisibility in some spaces, contributing to an identity that was always trying to be accepted.

———

"Show a people as one thing, only one thing, over and over again, and that is what they become."—Chimamanda Adichie

During my lifetime, I have experienced a world where Claire Huxtable exists both in the media and in real life; however, I have also been exposed to an imbalanced flow of sound bites and images that present distorted and broken representations of black women. Aside from the hypersexualized images that objectify black women, we have also been presented as people who are not in control of our own emotions and usually resort to aggressive attitudes or physical lash-outs when confronted by stress or trauma. Not only does this incomplete narrative illustrate a story that is imbalanced, but it also begins to construct the illusion that this is our only reality. Images become internalized, thus creating our reality based in incompleteness.

Even as I move through my second decade of practicing yoga and teaching in communities, my body is still questioned and challenged by those who are not accustomed to seeing full body types similar to mine move in certain ways. I regularly post photos and videos of myself moving through yoga postures on various social media platforms, and I often receive comments on how impressive my "stripper moves" are from both men and women. It is not my intention here to paint a picture that presents yoga as being any better or any worse than stripping; however, the truth is I am not stripping, I am practicing yoga. Comments like these contribute to a discourse that objectifies black and brown female bodies in a way that not only dehumanizes us, but views us through a sexualized lens that I seldom see used on white and thin female bodies that practice yoga. Similar to the critiques placed on my body as a young gymnast and later as a cheerleader, I continue to encounter reminders that my body may always be questioned. My yoga practice teaches me acceptance in that my body is not an inconvenience or a burden, but rather an opportunity to reclaim my position in any space I choose to occupy.

"Caring for myself is not self-indulgence, it is self-preservation, and that is an act of political warfare."—Audre Lorde

I never imagined that my yoga practice could be used as a tool for resistance. For many, it may seem contradictory to view a practice typically associated with peace and solace as a tool to confront racism, sexism, and other forms of oppression. My yoga practice makes me more aware and pushes me to ask why people who have been traditionally marginalized across multiple communities remain invisible throughout the pages of international yoga magazines. My yoga practice pushes me to resist the urge to make myself small as a black woman when I get flak for calling out racism. My yoga practice strengthens my ability to see myself in others and know that the same insecurities I had as a little black girl may resonate with the white guy next to me in class who has struggled with an eating disorder too. Yoga teaches me oneness and acceptance, not just within myself, but in ways that connect me to others as well.

I never want to give the impression that I have all of the answers, that I no longer experience pain, or that I do not still fight insecurity. I still have days when I look in the mirror and recognize that young girl who was never completely satisfied with her appearance. I still have moments in my life when my dress size fluctuates and my mind tries to seductively convince me I need a juice fast. There are days when I do not want to practice yoga; however, what is different is that I now have the tools that remind me that I am enough in every moment.

The people I meet through my work on *Chelsea Loves Yoga* and within communities inspire me to share my story and strengthen my journey to wholeness. I conduct a summer yoga camp for teen girls in Atlanta, Georgia, where teens practice yoga, read poetry, create literature, and rely on one another to process their lived experiences. I am inspired by the amount of courage these young women have as they utilize their yoga practice to confront their insecurities, think critically about the world, and cultivate self-love. Discussions that interrogate the portrayal of black women in the media followed by a Warrior series *asana* practice are reflected upon in their daily journals. A space has been established where realities are not ignored and swept under the rug just because they are uncomfortable to discuss.

My journey continues each day. Each day is an opportunity to practice something I learned on my mat in the world. Each day is an opportunity to connect more fully with myself in order for me to connect with others. Each day is an opportunity for me to love myself despite all of the things that tell me not to. My ability to use yoga as a way to connect, especially with our youth, gives me an opportunity to love my younger self in a way I was not capable of doing. Not because I didn't want to, but because I simply did not have the tools I needed to resist all of the outside messages that were influencing the image I had of myself. Through my yoga practice I am learning that in the acceptance of myself, I will continue to resist all that tries to take me further from the Self. My yoga practice is my acceptance and my resistance. I am enough.

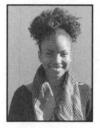

Chelsea Jackson is an Atlanta-based educator, blogger, and yoga instructor who works closely with teen girls. Chelsea is a PhD candidate at Emory University and founder of Yoga, Literature, and Art Camp for teen girls at Spelman College. Through her blog *Chelsea Loves Yoga*, she loves sharing the images and stories of yoga practitioners who have traditionally been silenced. www.chelsealovesyoga.com

Author photo by Valerie C. Jackson.

FINDING AND LOVING THE ESSENTIAL SELF

Alanis Morissette

What follows is a conversation between coeditor Melanie Klein (MK) and Alanis Morissette (AM).

MK: Anna and I are thrilled to have you share your story and wisdom, Alanis. We were compelled to write about the connection between body image and yoga for many reasons. One of them is because so often we hear the rhetoric "Love your body," but without providing practical tools to teach people how to do so, it's just an empty slogan. The practice of yoga has been a tool that we've been able to use over and over again in creating a new relationship to our bodies and body image, one that is gentler, kinder, and more forgiving.

You were a natural fit for this project from its inception. Not only are you a longtime practitioner, but you've been a vocal and adamant body image activist and an advocate for women's rights. We've been moved by your open and honest writing and your commitment to action.

Can you start by telling us about your relationship to your body in girlhood?

AM: My relationship to my body as a young girl was pretty sweet and untainted. I loved sports and was always trying to keep up with the boys on an athletic level; I very much enjoyed being a superjock.

MK: So you were the quintessential tomboy?

AM: I was—and playing sports had a positive impact on my body image. My body was a vehicle for movement and expression. It was empowering for me to use my body as an instrument rather than just being an ornament or decorative object. My body could *do* some exciting things!

MK: That's fabulous. There's definitely a positive correlation between sports and the self-esteem of girls. What kinds of sports were you playing?

AM: I played basketball, volleyball, and soccer—and I loved to play. Eventually, I also entered competitive swimming and was training at six in the morning seven days a week. I would swim, swim, and swim. Later I was invited to play baseball and there was also a potential scholarship as a pitcher. I definitely had this idea that I was going to be an athlete.

MK: So you spent most of your childhood immersed in the world of competitive sports?

AM: Yes, but I also was obsessed with the idea of dancing, dancing of any kind—from jazz and modern to tap. I realized I could move in a way that was entertaining to me while moving my blood and getting the endorphins going.

But dance presented me with challenges to my otherwise positive relationship with my body. One of the first challenges came when the comparative commentary that is so common in dance began. These negative comparisons taught me that there was a standard of how to dance, move, and look. I didn't quite get that standard consciously until I started being compared to other dancers. The thrill of moving my body and the pure, essential qualities being expressed were now being labeled and critiqued. It was hurtful and confusing.

MK: I bet. You came from a place of joy about being in your body to being taken out of your body and viewed as an object. How did that impact your dance obsession and your relationship to your body?

AM: It was devastating, and eventually dancing wasn't fun anymore. I stopped dancing when I was 12. The violence of the labeling, the competition, and the comparisons to a one-dimensional standard isn't just in the world of dance, though. It's everywhere in our culture. This is just when and where it started to encroach for me and enter my field of vision.

MK: You said you stopped dancing at 12 because of the negative climate, but that age is also associated with the onset of puberty for many girls.

AM: Yes, puberty was definitely a game changer for me. As I began to turn into a woman, I started gaining a few pounds and my hips started getting rounder. There are advantages to being like a boy in patriarchy, and up until then, I could play with the boys—I *was* "one of the boys." As a tomboy, my femininity was obscured and I was included. The boys would invite me to play hockey with them. I'd get the basketball in with a swish and walk around high-fiving everyone. Not only was I included and playing with the boys, I was good.

MK: How did you feel about puberty's changes on your body?

AM: There was a certain negativity that started around puberty and extended into the idea of becoming a woman. To me, the idea of moving away from what was a really androgynous approach to life into a more aesthetically and physically feminine body was terrifying. And I was not playing with the boys anymore. I wasn't invited because I was the girl all of a sudden.

MK: So your newly developing body, your curved feminine form, was essentially the cause of getting kicked out of the boys' club that you enjoyed and excelled within?

AM: Exactly—and I was bummin'.

MK: One of the things that makes your body image story unusual is your role in the world of entertainment—emerging as a young woman into the scrutiny of the public eye. Can you tell us when music and the larger entertainment industry entered your world?

AM: I was both a sensitive and precocious child and began writing music when I wasn't playing sports or dancing. I formed my own record label when I was 10, because unlike now, companies were not inclined to sign children to their labels.

MK: (laughs) Wow! You *were* precocious—there were potential scholarships for baseball on the line and you were writing music and forming record labels simultaneously.

AM: Entertainment and athletics were both so lovely to me that I never thought that I'd have to pick, but then at some point there's only so much time in the week.

MK: You chose music, obviously.

AM: Yes, I chose music, and by the time I was 16, my career went full-throttle in Canada and I was thrust into the scrutiny of the public eye.

MK: Aside from the negative comments in dance, was this the first time you experienced anything like this?

AM: To that magnitude, yes but the negative scrutiny started to happen even before I became highly visible. As you know, girls and women are constantly observed and critiqued in the culture from every angle. With the onset of puberty, I was no different—I was sexualized, objectified, and coincidentally no longer playing sports. At that point, I began to experience bullying comments about my body and started to scrutinize myself in my own head.

This was only exacerbated once I became a potentially marketable public commodity. I was told that if I wanted to be successful in the music industry, I would have to watch my weight and what I ate. It was devastating, especially since I had never gotten that feedback before. I was outright told that if I didn't eat less I would never succeed. It was only then, while my body was changing and I was growing into my femininity, that I was getting feedback like this.

MK: How did these comments and critiques of your body ultimately impact you, especially as you did emerge as a rising star and your visibility increased?

AM: Well, I went from being underweight to average weight, maybe a little higher. But I quickly learned from my producers, my managers, my peers, and the magazines I read that a tiny 12-year-old body was what the beauty standard was, and I no longer fit that ideal.

I was surrounded by some intense so-called mentors and people who wanted to exploit my gifts and talents, even if how I felt and my natural development needed to be trampled on in order to do that. The unsolicited feedback about my weight and food intake severely impacted my self-esteem and my relationship with food. They'd order a pizza, but I wasn't allowed to eat. I could order coffee, but I couldn't have cream.

Every version of hunger known to humankind came up for me. I felt like I had a hole in my being—I was always hungry: hungry emotionally, hungry for touch, hungry for mirroring, hungry for guidance that took my well-being into account, and I was hungry physically. Not only did I enter a state of anxiety, but my response was to eat alone and secretively, by the light of the fridge at four in the morning—only to be admonished for it the next day.

Upon sunrise, during professional trips with people I would work and travel with, I would hear the fridge open and I would hear rustling through the packages. They would monitor and count everything that had been in there the night before and everything I had eaten. I was shamed and scolded like a child. I felt like I was bad, wrong, and that my natural impulse could not be trusted. I felt my body and my appetite couldn't be trusted. I felt out of control and undisciplined, which ran counter to how strong-willed I was, and the high work ethic I had. I was a bad, bad, bad girl. This was never about my health; it became a measure as to whether I was "good" or "bad." But the biggest message was that I couldn't trust myself—the most dangerous message to send anyone.

I swung back and forth between anorexia and bulimia on the pendulum of eating disorders. I would gain a ton of weight by binging, binging, binging. Then I would realize I couldn't do this, and I would restrict and my weight would drop drastically in a worrisomely short period of time.

MK: Did anyone call you out on these rapid and severe fluctuations in your weight?

AM: No. Unchecked, my cycle of binging and restricting happened quickly and was fueled by my drive, a sense of perfectionism that is epidemic in this culture, and the dollars and livelihoods that were riding on it. Plus it provided me with a false sense of power and control. I couldn't control the chaos, but I could control the number on the scale. Control was the only mode of operation I could rely on. What do I have to do to get approval and get you all to calm the fuck down? What do I have to do? Lose 10 pounds? Okay, fine. I'll go and do that. I'd go and restrict and exercise. I needed the control because I had been taught and believed that I couldn't trust myself.

MK: How did you eventually overcome this incredibly dangerous and dysfunctional cycle, especially since you were in an industry that enabled and encouraged this sort of behavior?

AM: As soon as I got my license, I started to drive myself to therapy sessions in secret. I had looked in the yellow pages for a therapist I could afford, and I paid them from the money I earned from being on a television show as a 12-year-old.

MK: Wow—that's amazing and rare. To think that a young woman of your age and in your situation had the will and foresight to seek out professional help.

AM: I didn't think twice about speaking to someone who could be a teacher and provide some semblance of objectivity and a capacity to mirror some wisdom.

MK: And the therapy helped, obviously.

AM: Yeah, and I was reading everything I could get my hands on that would help me stop sticking my fingers down my throat. I read books like *The Cinderella Complex: Women's Hidden Fear of Independence* by Colette Dowling, and *Fat Is a Feminist Issue: The Anti-Diet Guide for Women* by Susie Orbach, and *Making Peace with Food: Freeing Yourself from the Diet/Weight Obsession* by Susan Kano. Intellectually, I was equipped to handle my eating disorder.

And I did get a handle on it, but there was still all this unconscious stuff playing out that the therapy helped with. There was a pause button pressed on the cycle of restriction and binging, but there was still a lot of anxiety—anxiety about being on display, and about being on the receiving end of judgment and envy.

With the release of my album in the United States, I went full circle. In many ways, I returned to the tomboy of my youth, which had provided a sense of a solace for me. Androgyny has always saved my life. In essence, I went back to the original gangster, who I always was.

MK: Ah, so this was around the time when *Jagged Little Pill* was released and you appeared in the "You Oughta Know" video with your leather pants and long hair. I mean, I couldn't even see your face in that video. You definitely didn't fit into the conventional female boxes of pop culture and the video genre of the time. I'll always remember how deeply those images of you impacted me at the time—the angst, the anger, the challenge to stereotypical images of women and female bodies. Needless to say, I was inspired. When did yoga enter the picture for you?

AM: Being on tour, bombarded with bright lights and workaholism, I needed to find a way to rejuvenate and move. I couldn't go to the gym and work out. In fact, I couldn't even leave my hotel room without being reacted to. Erich Schiffmann's VHS tape was perfect. Yoga was physical and peaceful—and I could do it in my hotel room by myself. God bless Ali McGraw.

MK: Given your history of playing sports and dancing, how did yoga make you feel and how did it impact your relationship to your body?

AM: I felt amazing doing yoga, and I was all in. In 1995, I began going to group classes regularly at Yoga Works on Montana Avenue in Santa Monica. People were tweaking out when I came to classes and workshops, but I was hell-bent on being a human being. This regular practice became a piece of my larger journey of awareness and introspection. I felt empowered. This was something only for me, not something that would be exploited or commoditized. Yoga offered a sense of reclamation of my spiritual practice, which had gone the way of all things after I lost faith in my Catholic upbringing. It provided ritual and became my prayer when I practiced alone—and the addict in me loved the high and the shaman in me loved the aesthetic.

But it took me fifteen years to actually truly be practicing yoga. Without a certain approach, it's so easy to use yoga as just another way to beat yourself up. As an extremist with an addictive personality, I would immerse myself in yoga and then be gone. Like with everything else, I would go full throttle. Then I would either be in pain or it would turn into sheer drudgery. So I would leave for a time and then return.

I knew it was a slippery slope and I saw the writing on the wall—I would be the girl who nailed the second series of Ashtanga and hurt herself. It takes a sophisticated spiritual journeyer to be able to appreciate what yoga is actually offering and I wasn't sophisticated enough. It was alluring; I knew there were elements in it that were going to be beneficial on many levels, and I was definitely infatuated with it. I felt strong. But it took a special teacher to help me reach the next level and make the practice my own.

MK: And who was that teacher?

AM: My twin brother, Wade. He started practicing yoga when I did, and once he did, he dove in. He went everywhere, including India, and learned as much as he could from every teacher he resonated with. Eventually, he started instructing me one-on-one and then I really got it. I became his student and he helped me make the practice my own. He was the first person to give me feedback about my practice. Most people ignored me because they were uncomfortable about my being a celebrity. He was the first person to tell me I had a "beautiful practice." I was so touched by this as I had felt my own practice, as well as my own life, was happening in an ignored vacuum. I began integrating different styles of yoga—with Ashtanga as the platform, I started learning about Iyengar and Krishnamacharya and Kundalini. And I loved all of it. I didn't judge who was "more legit" than anyone else. I developed a very intimate and personal relationship with my own practice. I'd be touring and writing music, and Wade would be out there learning. He is a very brave student-naturally-turned-teacher. Then he would meet me on tour and help lead my practice. I'd be in Slovenia doing a show and he would be there with the mat backstage. I was able to create my own space without being exploited or critiqued. He had seen my whole journey as an athlete, as his twin, as a yogi.

MK: Amazing—so yoga provided you that safe place of inquiry free from scrutiny you experienced everywhere else.

AM: Yes, exactly, and I began to inquire on the mat. If I was using it as another way to beat myself up, it was just another opportunity to inquire. Why am I doing yoga today? Do I want to be doing this? Why would I push through that pain? Why would I avoid it? And the ability to inquire in that way and stop, if need be, was a gift I learned from my brother. He was merciful with me because I had, not coincidentally, attracted teachers up to that point who were very masculine and "push-through" oriented. This was the only way I knew how to approach life. I went to yoga for a yin experience, and certainly I would hear the beautiful, pithy pull quotes that they would be saying, but at the same time I would be on the mat with them and have an altogether different experience. And it's painful because these people are teachers and yet I am not feeling loved, uplifted, inspired, or called to my highest. I was being pushed, in a way that felt antifeminine.

MK: I think that is beautiful—that your yoga practice evolved with the help of your brother. In fact, it seems he helped you discover the essence of yoga, in its purest form. How is your practice today?

AM: Things have changed. I am older, I'm on my way to being a bonafide crone—ha! As a person who is recognizable, as a wife and a mother,

I find I don't go to group classes that much. I'm learning to take better care of myself and listen to what I need. Sometimes I practice alone in our house; sometimes I practice with my brother or my friends. I like my own quiet experience and the kind of practice that my body dictates that day. I have a new sense of insight, awareness, and curiosity about my body, and now I have a practice that's tailor-made for me. Each time I'm on the mat, it's a different practice.

And while I have fine-tuned my understanding of yoga and its history and application, I still have moments of disassociation, moments when I think, "Whoa, I was really off there—that wasn't what I actually needed." But the commitment to growing my mindfulness is there.

Yoga is an approach to life for me. It's multifold. How can yoga not include everything? Because it *is* everything—my perfectionism that day, my exhaustion, my prowess, the gymnast in me—and it includes all the shadows. The evidence of whether I am forcing anything, or overly flexible, or attempting to ignore pain, or nurturing my body. Yoga is physical and spiritual. It's an attunement to all parts of me; it's the unity of being a whole person from my bones, muscles, and ligaments to my heart and intellect. And in touching every aspect of life, it includes the yin aspect of life and being: that part was revelatory for me. As soon as the restorative approach of yoga came into play, I recognized this is actually really feminine. I had always equated yoga, especially in my 20s, with the super-masculine. In the end, it's about what you need, having that self-knowledge enough to know what that is—discovering the true meaning and practice of moderation, and feeling connected to what is needed or wanted in any given moment.

As with my tendency toward extremism with sports, dance, food, and music, yoga had not always connotated moderation. It connotated extremism for me in the mid-nineties because that was the lens I was looking through. Moderation is a sure sign of evolution and self-care and maturation. These days, I have a more mature version of yoga in my mind and body. The paradigm shift took a long time. But once it began to shift, things began to soften and fall into balance, and I felt more equanimous in general, and definitely on the mat.

MK: Not only does that paradigm shift take time, it takes work. Changing our deeply ingrained perception of ourselves doesn't happen overnight. It can be challenging and exhausting, but it's ultimately worth it. Who doesn't want to feel peaceful and equanimous in their body and their life?

AM: Right—it's a process that takes work and attention, a constant evolution and inquiry. Yoga is a dear friend, and I have a tremendous respect for the practice. It's a great servant that shows up and asks what's happening now. What do you need now? For a long time I thought I had to fit my life into yoga, but it's the other way around. When I am in marathon training mode, I have a different yoga practice. When I just had a baby and I was experiencing postpartum depression, I had another practice. When I am on tour and running around stage like crazy and my brother is there, I have another practice. It's about integration and coming into wholeness and seeing, moment to moment, what is needed now.

All the parts are slowly coming together—into an integrated, connected, and woven-together state of balance. There's a sense of wholeness and a lack of apology for the essential self. There's this idealized woman I have been chasing at the cost of overlooking who I actually was the whole time, all along. I have more access to that and I am now surrounded, not coincidentally, with people who support that and love that about me as opposed to ignoring, judging, and rejecting those parts of me. I am less fragmented, and what I am having reflected back to me is less fragmented, more loving. More tender. And not a moment too soon.

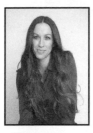 **Alanis Morissette** is one of the most influential singer-songwriter-musicians in contemporary music. Her albums have sold 60 million copies worldwide, as well as won her seven Grammys and the UN Global Tolerance Award. Outside of entertainment, Alanis is an avid supporter of female empowerment, as well as

spiritual, psychological, and physical wellness. She has contributed her writing and music to a variety of outlets and forums and causes, as well as running a marathon for the National Eating Orders Association and working with Equality Now. Alanis leads workshops and shares speaking/music engagements and keynote speaking worldwide. www.alanis .com

Author photo by Stuart Pettican.

PART FOUR

Parenting and Children

This section widens the lens from how yoga affects individuals' body image to how it can also support parents, parenting, and children. From this perspective, we start to see the effect that yoga can have on families and communities—which speaks to its power of transformation.

Kate McIntyre Clere gets us started with a provocative question: How does a mother support her daughter in navigating her way through a world of, at best, mixed messages about what it means to be a woman? Her fascinating answer—to reclaim the media through her own contribution—asks us to consider how yoga can be part of that conversation as well.

Next, Claire Mysko reflects on the many negative and conflicting messages that women receive about their bodies when they're pregnant, and how yoga helped her make her way through that with more balance. She wraps up with the potential of prenatal yoga to support women through their pregnancy in a positive way and how it can be part of a larger body image conversation.

From there, Dr. Dawn M. Dalili shares how yoga brought her back to her body, particularly during her pregnancy and as she became a parent. Using her background as a naturopathic physician, she also discusses how yoga can be part of a holistic approach to body image.

Finally, Shana Meyerson shares her experience and expertise as a yoga teacher for children. She offers stories from her teaching of how very early body image concerns come up for children of all genders, and how yoga can be part of what helps them both stay connected with and feel better about their bodies.

MOTHER VS. MEDIA

Kate McIntyre Clere

Help!

I am looking for ways to guide my 9-year-old daughter through the ubiquitous and invasive media landscape that undermines, sexualizes, trivializes, and bombards her every turn.

Any advice?

From Homemade Jumpers to Diamanté Tops

In 1973, I was 9 years old. I was the youngest of four living with our parents in a seaside neighborhood surrounded by the New Zealand bush. We spent our days biking the streets, navigating through the wild reserves, hauling logs to build bush cubbies, sailing dinghies on the windswept harbor, and building fires on the rocky foreshores. There was very little TV for children in New Zealand at the time, and in the evenings we would sit together and watch the one black-and-white TV channel with shows including *The Mary Tyler Moore Show*, *I Love Lucy*, and *The Brady Bunch*. Life for me was an endless adventure and anything was possible.

Fast-forward forty years to urban Sydney. Now my own beloved 9-year-old daughter, Miro, catches the bus to school and is exposed to hundreds of images of Photoshopped women on her journey. She loves to sing, dance, and watch music videos that have women portrayed as everything from superwoman to sex slave. Miro and I shop at the local mall where handbags, earrings, high-heeled shoes, padded bras, and diamanté tops are all marketed to 9-year-olds. Magazines covers flash sex, diets, plastic surgery, drugs, how to be hot for your man, creating a common language for my daughter and her friends. In the city there is hardly a moment of free air, space, or time when girls and women are not facing images of women that are digitally enhanced to an advertising executive's idea of perfection. So much has changed. So much now for my 9-year-old to deal with, let alone her mother.

Lost in the Media Maze

The pressure is on and I'm not sure I have the answers. I am often overwhelmed by the responsibility of guiding her through this bizarre maze of influences and feel ill equipped to dodge all the media images that do nothing to affirm Miro's unfolding girlhood or my life as a woman. Rather than running away to live somewhere free of these influences (if that place even exists), I want to help her learn to navigate them. It feels like a daily battle of "mother vs. media." Who can have the most influence? Family psychologist Steve Biddulph in his book *Raising Girls* says, "The mechanism of advertising is to attack your mental health—to worry you. If you want to sell products to a girl, whether she is four or fourteen, you first have to make her insecure—about her looks, friends, clothes, weight, skin, hair, interests, family, or ability. TV magazines, billboard, music, videos, and shopping malls pour this toxic message onto girls wherever they look."[1]

So how is this affecting us? Eighty percent of American women are dissatisfied with their body image.[2] When I first heard these figures, I knew we women were in the midst of an unspoken epidemic. What do we have to protect ourselves and our sense of self-worth from this undermining climate? This uncertainty is also affecting our daughters and their self-esteem. According to the National Survey of Young Australians, concern about how their body looks is now the biggest worry for the nation's 11- to 24-year-olds, with a recent report finding one in five 12-year-old girls regularly used fasting and vomiting to lose weight.[3]

Finding My Way Through

How are we as a society dealing with this ongoing issue? Are we even acknowledging the damage we are doing to our daughters? In my own search for meaning, one of the best ways I have found to connect with myself through the complexities of life is yoga. Through thirty years of life's challenges—the darkest days, losing loved ones, facing my fears, falling in love, giving birth, finding boundaries, growing up—it has always been yoga I turned to. Yoga has been and remains my closest ally, greatest teacher, champion, soothing soul mate, and toughest mirror. Yoga has been an integral part of my adult life and plays a prominent role in supporting my feminist perspective.

My classic yoga class scenario is rushing to get there, caught in my to-do list, still answering texts and wondering if I have the time for yoga today. Wondering if I am enough, if I deserve to focus on myself, pushing and pushing. Then, slowly, the miracle of yoga begins to unfold. I return to the breath, draw inside, and I find there on the mat lies that same childhood experience of freedom and possibility. In my experience, this clarity of self is the root of my feminism, allowing me to feel equal, valuable, and vital. The creative power and intuitive wisdom that arise naturally from my yoga practice are at the heart of my own self-worth.

So with that great image, one might imagine that I am serenely at ease with my own beauty, power, and worth. Sadly, no. This is not the case. I have been doing yoga for most of my adult life and still regularly confront my own self-worth. When did this dis-ease slip into my world? I feel the avalanche of the "perfect" looking, unempowered women in the media, and it cuts deep even when I am conscious of its incessant drive to promote insecurity. It would seem that while we can cut through that illusion and experience our own sense of self-worth through yoga, it's not something that you master then never have to address again. Like all disciplines, it takes consistent practice.

Through regular practice we can learn to rewrite our habits, breathe warmth around the incessant voice of the inner critic, and bring a consciousness to our daily lives. A regular yoga practice can ease the insecurities we harbor and gradually dissolve self-deprecating, distracted habits so we don't pass these insecurities on to our daughters.

Watching Mom

My plan is to raise my daughter so she is strong, vulnerable, valued, free, and secure, and does not have to spend serious amounts of her conscious and unconscious life hankering over her own body image and self-worth. How to do this? I think you start by changing the language, bringing a conscious and critical eye to the media, challenging the capitalist business model devoid of all ethics, and, most importantly, finding times and rituals to value the inner world. To create these positive neural pathways, I think the work is identical for both Miro and myself.

Girls are empathetic social creatures who watch their mothers' lives closely to help negotiate their own lives. From when Miro was quite young, I wanted to do what I could to prevent her from being burdened by or inheriting my insecurities. For example, I decided I would not linger in front of the mirror pointing out my faults. Rather, I decided to emphasize the positives and practice saying those out loud instead. (I do find it sad and numbingly boring that I can still have criticisms about my body after so many years!)

This decision to restrain what I give voice to is directly connected to the discipline of my yoga practice, and I see it as the yoga "working off the mat." Surrendering my mind and body to my daily yoga practice and moving through the *asanas* has gradually created a foundation of self-acceptance. Now when I am doubting myself, wondering if I am enough—angry, jealous, lost, and vulnerable—I first notice a physical response of dis-ease. From there, I am in a position to decide "where to from here?" What is the most loving, life-fueling way forward? Repeatedly noticing and returning to the present creates a more enlightened way of living, a clarity that can then inform all our choices.

These are valuable tools we can pass on to our daughters and I pass on to Miro: the practice of self-nurturing, mindfulness, and choice. I believe at 9 the most innate teaching I am giving my daughter is through modeling behaviors or even saying my own thoughts out loud, like, "I am not feeling great about my body this morning. I don't feel so great about wearing my bikini today. You know, Miro, sometimes my mind really believes these thoughts and it makes me feel really bad. So then I have to say to myself, it's okay. Bodies change shape all the time. I've got a choice and I'm not going to let these thoughts ruin my day at the beach. Let's go and enjoy ourselves!"

Weighing Our Food Choices

I feel very fortunate to live in a country where the quality and quantity of fresh and healthy food are abundant. However, with the pressure from the media for the perfect body, I see that food has sadly become another issue that can affect our sense of self-worth. In America, about ten million women and girls now battle with eating disorders such as anorexia and bulimia nervosa.[4] Although always a healthy eater myself, I have found that raising my daughter has encouraged me to be more awake to my own eating and become a mentor for her. I try to consciously observe when I am eating for hunger or to stifle feelings, and make an effort to find other ways to respond.

I was interested to come across the term "thin-heritance," newly coined from a study done in the UK. They found that "Teenage girls whose mothers diet are nearly twice as likely to have an eating disorder."[5] Women whose mothers dieted on and off throughout their childhoods remember cupboards filled with diet products, calorie counting, and anxious attitudes around food. A mother's dieting and low self-image permeate her children's own eating habits and self-image issues well into adulthood.

Getting really clear on our food values and connecting more consciously to food is an important skill we can pass on to our daughters. For me, this awareness of diet is woven throughout my life of yoga— not only in the literature but also in my own experience. Regular yoga practice heightens my awareness of my dietary choices, the respect I have for food, the response my body has to food, and the state I am in when eating. As a family, we choose a vegetarian diet and often discuss the ethics of what we eat and the food industry. In yogic literature, it is written that some foods "create new energy, clarity, and a clear, calm mind, enabling us to use all our mental, physical, and spiritual abilities" and that other foods can disturb either our physical or emotional balance: "Too much of these foods can cause restlessness, agitation, and a distracted mind." [6] By observing my own reaction to foods, I have come to know more clearly what best suits my body and what time of day I should be eating—and my daughter witnesses all this. Miro often asks questions like, "Why don't you want a doughnut, they're so yummy?" I say, "Yeah, when I was a kid I loved them, but you know, now I notice that they don't make me feel so great. I feel better if I eat an apple. You'll get to know what food makes you feel happier."

Passing on the Perfect

I am already feeling the pressure to be the perfect mother. So much literature says we, as mothers, are the most influential person in our daughters' lives, and as I type this I see my faults arising! All around us we see media images of perfect women, with perfect figures, in perfect clothes, raising perfect children, who maintain perfect households, perfect manners, and are perfect conversationalists—oh, and who are perfectly sexy as well!

The ongoing comparison that draws us away from our inner wisdom can manifest into depression or anxiety. Trying to be perfect makes me stressed. It makes me impatient with my kids. I respond angrily when I am feeling out of control, when I am late, the dinner is burning, my clothes aren't coming together, I did not remember to buy food for school lunches, etc.

Breathing, deep breathing learned and practiced in meditation and on the mat is my only cure here. Knowing how to take a pause and reflect. Noticing the racket. Recognizing the symptoms of overwhelm, shame, tiredness. Letting the kids know how I am feeling, acknowledging I am unable to do the things we had planned, being open with them, practicing self-compassion. It's my hope that being open with Miro will support her in being honest and compassionate with herself if or when she finds herself in the grip of thoughts and feelings that steal her from her self-accepting heart.

Imagining Ourselves into Being

As a teenage girl, I saw media images of women in stereotypical roles as housewives and homemakers. A woman was subservient, and her purpose was primarily to please her man and care for her family. This image never sat well with me, and I was clear from about the age of 16 that I would never become one of these women! I wanted choices; I would be the hero of my own life, free to discover and fulfill my own unique destiny. Having the courage to listen to this response and to give space and energy to hear that authentic inner voice are some of the gifts of yoga. This feeling of connection is what I want to pass on to Miro. I want her to connect with her authentic nature. I want her to be free to find her passions.

More recently I am sorely challenged by trying to protect her from the deluge of sexualized images that come her way—the soft porn of billboard advertising, the overt sexuality of MTV, and the up-aging of clothing for her age group. Just when she is starting to look outside of herself for role models and mentors, the majority of media images of woman are nude or barely clothed, objectified, placid, male-pleasing, vacuous, skinny, and white. We haven't got to the world of Internet porn yet, but I am bracing myself for more and more explanations and ways to express a powerful connection with her own sexuality and choices. Where do our young girls find a safe, protected space to explore their emerging womanhood and imagine themselves into being?

Until recently, I've chiefly avoided commenting on skewed portrayals of women so as not to draw attention to them and create interest for Miro. However, I now see evidence with Miro and her friends that they are adapting their play to align with the media imagery they're exposed to. As they sing, dance, dress up, and play, I observe them role-playing as languid, pouting, and sexy sirens. I want to give Miro a chance to play a myriad of characters: strong warrior, princess, shaman, mother, or president. To balance the objectified images of women Miro encounters, I try to draw her attention to less publicized role models. In Sydney, we have a female mayor, governor, and prime minister, so we talk about what their lives are like and what they are able to achieve. I regularly voice my enthusiasm for women around us who are choosing lives they are passionate about.

YOGAWOMAN: *Creating a New Media Paradigm*

Every working mother I know struggles with the work/family balance. Keeping myself available for Miro's needs both physically and emotionally is always a challenge. One of the highlights of mixing my work with family was when we were creating our film *YOGAWOMAN*. Telling the stories of more than fifty strong, passionate yogis from around the globe created a three-year conversation at our home that celebrated women in all their magnificent stages of life. We created the film to highlight the ways in which women are using yoga to stand in their own power. Seeing these women portraying their real lives on the big screen was inspirational and offered women everywhere role models, inviting them all to be part of a community to build their own authentic voices. A radical counter to the mainstream media, our film offered ninety minutes packed full of wisdom and practical tools for creating a new paradigm together.

With the mat as our laboratory, there are so many things to discover about ourselves as we adapt through the different cycles of our lives. On the mat, in this quiet space, we see our habits, face our limits, feel our pain, and breathe through our edge of fear. This tool is invaluable for my life and for parenting. As a mother I often feel Miro's pain and desires as if they were my own. Instead of reacting, blaming, wanting to collude with her distress and become the victim of our circumstances, yoga has given me other responses to offer her. Together we practice leaning in to the experiences of life—pain, suffering, joy, failure, success—and learn that we are able to be in all these places and it's okay. There is always learning to be had from every circumstance, and with the breath as a tool, we can fully engage in all of life.

There are times I feel overwhelmed with the task of just trying to keep myself together, but I see clearly that being a mother has become part of my yogic practice. My learning is to stay on the "family mat," lean in to the challenges, and be present for this life-changing role. If I can help Miro build a sense of awareness of herself that is respectful, kind, compassionate, and self-accepting regardless of external media prompts and other outer biddings, I feel I will have done my job well as mother and attained something in my own passage to authentic womanhood.

1. Steve Biddulph. *Raising Girls*. New York: Harper, 2013.
2. L. Smolak. *National Eating Disorders Association/Next Door Neighbors Puppet Guide Book*. NEDA: 1996.
3. Justin Healy. *Body Image and Self-Esteem*. Thirroul, NSW, Australia: Spinney Press, 2008.
4. J. H. Crowther, E. M. Wolf, and N. E. Sherwood. "Epidemiology of Bulimia Nervosa" in M. Crowther, D. L. Tennenbaum, S. E. Hobfoll, and M. A. P. Stephens, eds., *The Etiology of Bulimia Nervosa: The Individual and Familial Context* (Washington, DC: Taylor & Francis), 1–26.
5. Jane Kirby. "Many Girls 'Damaged' by Their Mum's Dieting." *The Independent*, www.independent.co.uk/life-style/health-and-families/health-news/many-girls-damaged-by-their-mums-dieting-1811258.html (accessed March 2014).
6. Carol DiPirro. "What Is a Yogic Diet?" *My Yoga Online*, www.myyogaonline.com/healthy-living/nutrition/what-is-a-yogic-diet (accessed March 2014).

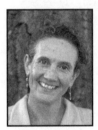

Kate McIntyre Clere cofounded Second Nature Films following a successful career as an actor and theater director. She is the coproducer, director, and writer of the award-winning film *YOGAWOMAN*, the world's first feature documentary about women and yoga. Throughout her adult life, Kate has practiced and taught yoga, bringing balance and strength into her roles as filmmaker, wife, and mother. www.yogawoman.tv

Author photo by Clara Gottgens.

TUNING OUT THE "BABY BUMP" MEDIA MADNESS: HOW PRENATAL YOGA HELPED ME FIND REAL BODY IMAGE BALANCE

Claire Mysko

The walk to my prenatal yoga class at the YMCA took me through Brooklyn neighborhoods full of brownstones and Bugaboos. I would cross the honking, blaring buzz of Flatbush and head over to Atlantic Avenue, where the spicy scents from the Middle Eastern shops quickly gave way to "artisanal" aromas wafting out of cafés selling overpriced coffee and scones freshly baked with locally sourced organic ingredients. It was a relief to be able to smell food and not immediately feel waves of nausea. My Summer of Ginger Beer was officially over. I had made it to my second trimester and the crisp fall air made everything feel fresh and full of possibility. I was expecting! I could finally ditch my don'tpukeohpleasedon'tpuke mantra and come up with something a little more cheerful and life affirming. This was all kinds of awesome.

On that trek, which I made twice a week for the remainder of my pregnancy, I would pass by a tiny magazine shop. It was bigger than a sidewalk newsstand but not big enough to offer much of a selection. No artsy titles or imports, but they had all the tabloids. Propped up in the window, the headlines read: *"Baby bump or too many burritos?" "Pregnancy cravings revealed!" "How she got her body back after baby!"* I had just finished coauthoring a book about how our culture's obsessive fixation on weight before, during, and after pregnancy is profoundly damaging to women and, by extension, to our children. I had spent months in the role of "body image expert," interviewing women about their personal stories. And now I was preggo.

As a recovering perfectionist with a history of disordered eating, I was determined not to stress about having the perfect pregnancy. I wasn't going to drive myself nuts ruminating over whether it was okay to get a pedicure (the chemicals!) or how much I should scale back on my cappuccinos (the caffeine!). But there were some toxins I did stress about—the toxins that caused nearly 80 percent of the women my co-author and I surveyed for our book to say that the fear of gaining weight and not being able to lose it after delivery was their *number one* body-related pregnancy concern. I knew there were specific things I could do to protect myself from being in that 80 percent, so I did those things by the book—the book I wrote. I took my own advice and took weight out of the equation. I allowed my obstetrician to weigh me, but I never looked at or tracked that number myself. I continued to eat intuitively. I packed up my skinny jeans and pencil skirts soon after I saw that plus sign on the pregnancy test, lest I be triggered by the experience of trying to squeeze into anything when my body started rapidly expanding. I set boundaries with my nearest and dearest. I had a solid support system at the ready. I journaled. In an actual journal. Of course I couldn't plan for everything, especially living in a city like New York, home to high-end gyms that charge memberships equivalent to a mortgage and where the beauty-is-thinness mindset is so firmly entrenched that the images and messages are a daily assault to the senses. It quickly became clear that in order to have a body-positive pregnancy, I needed to bolster my inner resources and find a way to detox from the external pressures. My prenatal yoga practice served both purposes.

The Power of Doing

In every yoga class, I took a moment to survey the room filled with women at various stages of their pregnancies. Some, like me, teetered and swayed until they found their roots for tree pose. This was a space where the purpose was to find balance with our changing bodies. Struggle against the added weight and you will falter. It was a truth that steadied me inside the yoga studio, and in my life outside of it.

Pregnancy is a time when our bodies work some serious magic. Unfortunately, we're living in an environment where the hyper-focus on how we look—how much weight we gain, how we're dressing our "bumps," how we should be racing to get our bodies back as soon as that little bundle of joy arrives—can make it all feel a little less magical. The diet, fitness, fashion, and beauty industries have woken up to the fact that stoking women's prenatal and postpartum appearance anxiety adds up to mucho dinero. Enter the Spanx maternity collection and multimillion dollar contracts for stars such as Mariah Carey, who described her pregnant body as "rancid" and then became a spokesperson for Jenny Craig, and Jessica Simpson, who was publicly shamed and body-snarked for her pregnancy weight gain and soon after signed a contract that had her stepping on a Weight Watchers scale made of pure gold.

Pregnancy offers a valuable opportunity to tune in to our own power and tune out all the other B.S. Piles of research point to the fact that girls and women benefit from learning to appreciate what their bodies can do. This internal knowledge can steer us away from the dangerous path of valuing ourselves based on what we look like or what size we can fit into. For me, yoga was a visceral way to honor what my body was up to. At the start of class, the instructor asked each of us to share what was going on that week. One by one, the aches and pains would be revealed, the sleep disturbances aired, the milestones marked. And then we would move on to the practice of working with those bodies, in all their messy, baby-growing imperfections. For me, each movement was a purposeful move toward making peace, not waging war.

Breaking Out of Battle Mode

As women, we have learned to see our bodies as adversaries—entities to be conquered and controlled. We grow up hearing that dessert is sinful and that we should satisfy our every craving with fat-free yogurt. We absorb the lie that "thin and pretty" will get us a hell of a lot more in life than "strong and powerful." In a culture that makes it nearly impossible to feel confident in our bodies, it is perhaps not so shocking that 65 percent of American women admit to being disordered eaters.[1] Their behavior might not fit the diagnostic criteria for eating disorders such as anorexia, bulimia, or binge eating disorder, but their fixation on food and weight is a supremely negative force in their lives. Obsessive calorie counting, chronic dieting, over-exercise, and secret eating are some of the many damaging patterns that make up our national epidemic of disordered eating. And let's face it: if two-thirds of women fit somewhere on this spectrum, it stands to reason that a good number of us are or will become mothers. It would be a lovely Utopian fantasy to imagine that pregnancy would be a blissful respite from all the body pressures, a time to bask in some goddess-like glow that would eclipse all those nasty whispers of "not good enough." And you know what? For some women, pregnancy really *is* effortlessly like that. I swear. I have met these women. They've been lovely and wonderful and kind of awe-inspiring. I am not one of them.

I had been recovered from my eating disorder for over a decade when I first found out I was pregnant. I was in a pretty good place with my body image too. I had a few rough days here and there, but for the most part I felt solidly happy with the way I looked—it was a world of difference from the near-constant self-doubt I lived with for so many years. I had no way of knowing how or if pregnancy would upset that healthy balance I had worked so hard to reach. But if I wasn't going to feel like a glowing goddess (which I didn't), I wanted to make damn sure I didn't slip back into that dark, familiar place where I felt like utter crap about my body. So I let my body do what it was doing. I was okay with the transformations most of the time—and I let myself have moments of not being okay too. I made a promise to myself that I would reach out when I found myself on those "not okay" curves so that they would not turn into downward spirals. And they didn't. I realized that I was hardest on myself when I was most worn down by the stress of the scary "what if?" medical tests, the agony of being on the verge of puking from morning sickness (which is one of the world's most egregious misnomers, as mine was certainly not limited to the hours before noon), or the exhaustion that came from schlepping my pregnant ass all around town on NYC public transit. (People, look up from your iPhones! Offer a seat, for the love of all that is holy.) I tuned in to my real-life triggers, and I did my best to tune out the media messages that make it so easy for us to turn on ourselves. We are sold the idea that "managing" our appearance with products, food, and B-list-endorsed plans will help us manage the feelings and fears of pregnancy and new motherhood that often seem so messy, untenable, and—yes, I'll say it— shameful. We are not supposed to be vulnerable and freaked out about this enormous life event that will change nearly every aspect of our lives. But weight-conscious? Well, *of course* that's okay. In fact, it's expected.

Want to know the pregnancy-related buzz phrases that make my skin crawl the most? It's the insidious, oppressive directive to "get your body back." It's the obligatory laundry list of "how she did it" that accompanies every women's magazine profile of every celebrity who happens to have given birth within the last twenty-four months. It's the incessant onslaught of "post-baby bikini bodies." The reason these empty promises are so effective is because marketers and media makers have successfully identified that many women *do* experience a loss of who they are (you know, existential-style) when they make the move into the mother hood. And with dollar signs twinkling in their eyes, they have advertised and proselytized to the point where we are quick to believe that the key to regaining it is to lose the weight. It's not just our self-worth that has become tied up in what we look like—it's our very sense of self.

Being a media-literate mama has helped me keep my critical eyes open, especially when passing newsstands or clicking through guilty-pleasure entertainment blogs. Being in therapy has helped me talk it all out and work through the vulnerabilities that used to lead me to restrict, binge, or purge. It was my prenatal yoga practice that brought me to a place where my physical movement intertwined the threads of who I was with the person I was and am becoming. It's still, and always will be, a work in process. Yoga was decidedly and definitely not about weight I was gaining or when I would lose it.

Silence and Savasana

I'll say it. *Savasana* was my favorite part of the prenatal yoga package. Not just because I was so dead tired that the whole "corpse pose" thing made a whole lot of sense, but because the quiet of it sustained me. Pregnancy comes with an insane amount of noise—questions about our choices, expectations about who we should be and what we should look like.

The sirens are blaring: don't gain too much weight, eat this but not that, get your plan in place to take off the baby weight. And then the internal alarms kick in: I'm too smart, too feminist to be worrying about how my butt looks in maternity jeans. Holy crap, how will I protect my child from the body image struggles and eating disorders that ate up so many years of my life? The static is paralyzing, but we lose out if we just try to keep moving through it. Yoga taught me that the remedy is to find stillness, to listen to what silence will tell you. Lying on that cool, wood floor with the lights off, propped with more and more cushions as the months wore on, I would hear the breath of other women in the room, each of them facing their own onslaught of pressures. In and out. Some sighs. Some coughs. I was not alone. Later in my pregnancy, I would feel my baby—then my *daughter*—swimming around, her kicks and movement gloriously louder to me there in that room than in any other space. I was not alone.

Prenatal yoga was never a solitary practice for me. It was about connection, with the women around me and with my child. The ever-present messages about molding and shaping our bodies to meet some manufactured ideal are effectively disconnecting us from what really matters about pregnancy and motherhood. They disconnect us from each other too, keeping us far from the conversations that will move us to healthier place.

Imagine if instead of "You look great! You barely look pregnant! I wish I could have had such a cute little bump," we started with a simple "How are you?" That question framed my prenatal yoga experience. It was verbalized. It was internalized. It was practiced.

1. UNC School of Medicine. "Survey Finds Disordered Eating Behaviors Among Three Out of Four American Women." *UNC School of Medicine*, April 22, 2008, www.med .unc.edu/www/newsarchive/2008/april/survey-finds-disordered-eating-behaviors-among-three-out-of-four-american-women (accessed March 2014).

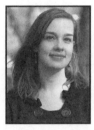

Claire Mysko is an award-winning author and an internationally recognized expert on body image, leadership, and media literacy. Her book for girls, *You're Amazing! A No-Pressure Guide to Being Your Best Self*, was named to the Amelia Bloomer List, a project of the American Library Association that recognizes outstanding feminist books for young readers. She is also the coauthor of *Does This Pregnancy Make Me Look Fat? The Essential Guide to Loving Your Body Before and After Baby*. www.clairemysko.com

Author photo by Kate Glicksberg.

RX: YOGA

Dr. Dawn M. Dalili

Have you ever gone through something challenging and thought to yourself, "I learned my lesson. I'll never do that again"?

The problem with this line of thinking is that many of our most important, and most challenging, life lessons require repeats (and sometimes three- or four-peats). Each time we go through them, we get the lesson a little bit deeper.

And so it was with my yoga practice.

This particular time, it was the fall of 2009. The blistering heat of the Arizona summer was barely beginning to ease, and I was returning to the mat after a long hiatus. The door to the studio opened and out poured the heat, steam, and potent odor of fifty-plus sweaty bodies that took the previous class. That familiar, pungent smell did not diminish my excitement for being back on the mat or in a studio. Waving my hand in front of my face to clear a path through the humidity as I walked into the room, I found the back corner where I suspected I would have a little more space and the air might smell fresher. The room slowly filled around me, and I was afforded the luxury of neither space nor fresh air.

I hadn't been in a studio for over three months, and I wasn't sure what to expect from this class. The last time I was on a mat I felt strong, powerful, beautiful, magical even. On this day, I was excited, nervous, giddy, anxious, and … to be honest, I was also tired and achy. My body didn't feel like my own.

After a few minutes, the teacher entered the room. The stereo was turned up; the lights were turned down and we started in child's pose. My hips creaked as I shifted my weight back, but it felt good to lean into them.

As I pressed into the first Down Dog, I remember thinking, "Isn't this a resting pose?!" My arms did not seem to have the strength required to support my body. My hips and hamstrings were too bound to let my legs participate in bearing the weight of this posture. My neck did not recall how to relax the tension ingrained in its fibers.

On this day, I was a beginner to the yoga practice—all over again.

The First Beginning

The first time I was new to yoga, I was almost ten years younger and my body was strong, even if my mind was a bit rigid and inflexible. I had entered the yoga studio reluctantly after a chiropractor suggested I stretch my hamstrings to prevent another back injury. Yoga was simply a means to an end. My objective was well defined and very specific. The goal was to improve my flexibility so that I could continue running.

I strongly identified as an athlete, and I was clear that I wasn't interested in any of the "hippy dippy bullshit" that came with meditation, chanting, or a spiritual practice. Out of sheer obligation, I returned to the mat three times a week to stretch and sweat—no more.

Am I Better Than Yesterday?

From the outside, my practice was innocent, benign even. I didn't levitate, nor did I contort my body in ways seen on magazine covers. I simply touched my toes without bending my knees. No one realized how I felt on the inside. At this point, I was still convinced that yoga, like all things in life, was about goals and objectives. Secretly thrilled by touching my toes, I gazed up to see if balloons were falling from the sky. They weren't.

However, what followed changed my practice and turned my life upside down.

"Now you can work on extending your spine and the inward spiral of your thighs." The instruction was simple: take the length, space, and experience you have created and create more length, more space, and a deeper experience.

For me, running had always been about two variables—speed and distance. I found comfort in activities with measurable outcomes. Daily, I looked at my run times to assess my progress. This was how I answered the question: "Am I better today than I was yesterday?" Days on which the answer was *no* were gloomy and filled with reproach.

When I was encouraged to explore spaciousness and length, it struck me as being vague. "I can't measure that!"

My world opened up. And my world fell apart.

My teacher's guidance opened doors that I instinctively knew led to more doors and, behind them, even more doors. She showed me that yoga was an ever-expanding path. The further along this path I traveled, the more of a beginner I would become. While balloons did not fall around me, on the inside there were fireworks! I began to question my reliance on measurable outcomes as an indication of my worth and the determinant of my well-being.

That night, I threw away my running shoes.

Not a Member of the Spandex Club

I exchanged my gym membership for a membership at a yoga studio and experimented with classes that incorporated chanting and meditation, but I was still attached to my image of what it means to be a yogi. That image was long, lean, flexible, and smokin' hot in spandex.

My body was bulky from twenty years of playing soccer and running. I couldn't do handstands and other arm balances, and I felt terribly self-conscious in spandex. I would sit before class and look around the room wondering if I would ever do the things I saw others doing. I wondered if

I would ever look the way the others looked. I bought into this idea that I had to eat a certain way and dress a certain way to be *yoga*.

I was convinced that yogis had their own exclusive club, and I was not a card-carrying member. I could pay to take classes, but I was simply an outsider looking in.

This belief changed slowly as I played around with smaller, quieter classes that naturally encouraged a more introspective and personal experience. I remember the day a teacher, whose class I was new to, whispered in my ear, "Consider that how it feels might matter more than how it looks." He often suggested that we do short sequences with our eyes closed, not to challenge our balance, but to go inward and *feel* the postures. When I closed my eyes, I felt a serenity I could not attain when watching and comparing myself to others.

Voted Off the Island?

I lived in San Francisco, so I had regular access to some of the world's most famous yoga teachers. Of course, their wisdom influenced my progress. But my three greatest teachers were the situations that forced me to begin my yoga practice again: a bike crash that cracked a rib and kept me from practicing for six weeks; a skiing accident that crushed my knee, required multiple surgeries to repair, and prevented me from walking for over three months; and pregnancy, a journey that changed everything about my body and my relationship to it.

Over the years of practicing, I was becoming more long, lean, and flexible like the others who took classes. Without noticing, I had become deeply attached to what my body could do. But these wise teachers forced me to see the ways I defined myself. When injured, I would panic. *Will I get fat? Will I lose my membership in this club?*

Each of these situations forced me to question all that I assumed about myself and yoga. Injuries and life changes moved me one step further from goals and measurable outcomes that marked my worth and one step closer to presence and acceptance of what is.

Yoga slowly became a platform for me to learn about me. My practice led to questions such as *Who am I? What do I feel?* and *What do I want out of life?*

Giving Birth to All That I Am

During pregnancy, I started to feel truly feminine for the first time in my life.

Growing up, I was all tomboy. I played soccer and climbed trees; if I wasn't covered in dirt, I wasn't happy. I felt grossly out of place in junior high when other girls gravitated toward cheer and dance and I still wanted to chase a ball. I didn't want to wear skirts, dresses, or makeup, but the pain of not fitting in was so palpable that my belly constricts as I type these lines today. It wasn't until I found yoga at the age of 21 that I began to explore a more feminine side of myself.

When I got pregnant, it had been more than ten years since I had last purged following a meal, and what I discovered is that I still viewed my body as something to shape and control. Having struggled with disordered eating and an eating disorder in my teens, my softness and curves were not a thing I welcomed. Just like when I got injured, when I found out I was pregnant one of my first fears was of getting fat.

And then one day, I felt him move. I felt the life within me, and I discovered my magic. I saw my body as a vessel that creates and supports life, and I let go of all my anxiety about weight and shape. I continued to practice yoga, but with an ease and softness I had not experienced before. My yoga practice became an exploration. It was for us, not me.

In forty-one weeks, I had gained roughly 55 pounds, and I've never felt more comfortable with food or my body. I felt confident. Strong. Womanly. Graceful.

My birth experience was equally affirming. My son was born at home with the help of my midwife. My mother was there to offer her support. After six intense hours, I held my son and, at the age of 30, learned the meaning of the word *love.*

I embraced the baby moon, as my midwife calls it, the four-week period of recuperation and bonding following the birth. I found humor in the weird things my body did, like spray milk when I was in the shower. I looked at the loose skin around my belly and considered it a comfy place for my son to lay his head during a nap. I remained caught up in the magic of the process. I was in awe over what my body had done and what it was doing to support and nourish this precious person. No amount of fatigue could rob me of the pride or joy that coursed through my system.

At the end of the baby moon, I wanted back on the mat. And slowly, like catching a cold, I began to have thoughts about wanting my pre-baby body back.

The Horror

Even though I didn't think it was possible, the yoga room on that crowded day got even hotter. My body warmed up, and the achiness faded. Perspiration collected at my brow. The salutations began to feel familiar, like catching up with a friend I hadn't seen in years. I slowly began to relax into the postures.

Twice my instructor gestured toward my belly and suggested I engage my core. "Isn't it engaged?" I thought as I glanced down at my navel, which stubbornly refused to respond to my greatest efforts to pull it up and in. "Why doesn't it move? Will it ever move?"

The mind chatter was off to the races, and I began to feel very self-conscious. "Should I be in spandex? ... Wow, look at her, she's beautiful ... Will my body ever do that again?"

About thirty minutes into the practice, as sweat dripped from my hairline and brow, my breasts began to leak. My shirt was soon damp but not with sweat. My milk was letting down.

Shame. Humiliation. Horror. If I could've wrapped myself in my mat and disappeared, I would have.

Beginning Again

Every time I held Everett in my arms, I remembered my magic. I felt spiritual in a different way than I had ever experienced, even in yoga and meditation. When I looked at my son, my connection to life could not be questioned.

In spite of that deep connection, I walked into the yoga studio and felt self-conscious, insecure, and fat. I completely lost touch with what, just moments earlier, felt beautiful, magical, and connected to the source of life. I couldn't complete classes without taking breaks. I couldn't do handstands or gracefully jump forward after Down Dog. My breasts, triple their pre-pregnancy size, got in the way of everything. I felt awkward and felt self-conscious about looking lazy.

But I was lucky. This was not my first experience as a beginner on the yoga mat. The first time, my body was strong and my mind was rigid. This time, my body was softer and so was my mind. I had the gift of ten years of slow, steady learning that culminated with my first experience of love.

Yoga taught me to look inward. I recalled the whisper, "Consider that how it feels might matter more than how it looks."

Yoga taught me to notice my judgments and get curious. In my first teacher training, I learned to fall back frequently on the phrase "Isn't that interesting!" Through yoga, I learned to stay present when tempted to distract myself from an uncomfortable experience. Yoga taught me to allow, especially when forcing proved to be so ineffective. Beginning again and again taught me that I am far more resilient than I had given myself credit for being.

Somewhere along the way, I had learned that I could only love another as much as I loved myself. Accepting this as truth, I realized that I must love myself as much as I love Everett.

Stepping back from the shame, stepping back from how I thought it looked to others, and stepping back from all the *shoulds* and *shouldn't*s with which I had been berating myself, I decided to extend myself the gift of love.

The next time I walked into the studio, I reassured myself that all those people doing handstands before class were more likely to be looking in the mirror at themselves than at me, so what did it matter if I modified every posture to suit myself? When I felt tired or discouraged, I pictured Everett and felt my connectedness to something much higher than I could ever comprehend. I traded nitpicking for embracing the new shape of my body.

My Yoga Mat, Myself

Did practicing yoga heal my body image or did my eventual acceptance of my body save my yoga practice? I may never know the answer to that question. What I do know is that yoga and my relationship with my body are intimately intertwined. My yoga mat is a safe place for me to be me; and at one time, it was the only place that felt safe for me to explore my relationship with my body and self. As I got comfortable with revealing myself on the mat, I was gradually able to extend my authenticity outward. My yoga practice has become where I discover my truth.

And that truth is not always beautiful. Sometimes, I get on the mat and find anger, frustration, sadness, and judgment. Other times, I find spaciousness, relaxation, and peace.

Yoga has opened a dialogue with my body. In these conversations, my body has taught me that no matter how hard I push, it will push back harder, giving me whatever reminder I need to listen to its needs, not what my mind *thinks* it needs. It is infinitely more efficient to ease up on the reins. My body has taught me that I will never be perfect, but it is always interesting to explore my beliefs around perfection.

Rx: Yoga

I have taken these lessons from the mat to heart, and I now apply them through the lens of being a naturopathic physician. I became a naturopath because I deeply resonated with the idea of practicing medicine that honored body, mind, and spirit. But my education left me with a deep understanding of body and little of mind and spirit. Fortunately, my mat has taught me the rest.

Herbs, supplements, a healthy diet, exercise, and well-placed acupuncture needles are useful in helping a body to heal, but they pale in comparison to time, patience, compassion, and acceptance. One's willingness to go inside, listen, and respond to the feedback a body provides is not just the key to a meaningful yoga practice; it is the key to a meaningful life.

Everett is now four, and since returning to the mat after pregnancy, I have had the opportunity to begin again a few more times. I have dropped my resistance to the process, recognizing that these great challenges are the doorway to life's greatest gifts.

My lessons on the mat, my lessons as a mother—and even more so, my lessons with starting over again and again—give me a unique depth of compassion as a doctor and mentor. My clients are frequently startled when I say, "That's great!" after they've come in telling me they've fallen off the wagon in one way or another. They are startled because they can see that I mean it. And it really *is* great! It is great because they showed up again. It is great because they are blessed with the opportunity to be a beginner again and to experience beginning with a newly informed perspective. It is great because they've learned something about how they face challenges.

I would never have been able to walk someone safely through their own learning process if it hadn't been for my own struggles with beginning again.

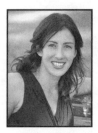

Dawn M. Dalili, ND, is a naturopathic physician licensed in the state of Arizona. She lives in northwest Florida with her son, where she teaches yoga and serves as a consultant on natural health and wellness. Dawn believes that health is often a reflection of a deeper sense of self, and she approaches health and wellness through the doorways of body image and self-worth. www.dawndalili.com

Author photo by Sherri Butler Photography.

"I'M UGLY! I'M SO UGLY!"

Shana Meyerson

I know a yogini (you may know her too ... she's pretty famous in the yoga world) who is as bendy as a rubber band, strong as an ox, and graceful as a swan. She also happens to know the sutras inside and out and, by all respects, is the epitome of the modern-day yogini.

She would be *such* a perfect cover model for any yoga magazine on earth. She is gorgeous and she's got curves. Don't read too much into this. I am not using the word "curves" as a euphemism for fat. She has a body that is strong but feminine. She's not a size 0; she *may* be a size 4. And according to a best-selling yoga publication, that's just too darn fat to grace their cover.

Funny, before I was told this, I never even realized that all of the yoga cover models are cute, petite, perfectly proportioned women. Before I heard this story, I would have told you that *anyone* could be a cover model if they were dedicated enough to their practice. I thought *I* could be on the cover some day. Right. No chance they would put my size 6 *tuchas* on their cover. Let me just say that if my strong penchant for desserts was ever a barrier to entry, it's a concrete barrier now.

By the way, let me take a moment to mention that while size 6 is smaller than the average American woman (who wears a size 14), it is still considered to be too large in the mainstream media culture. "Plus size" would be the exact term they use.

I guess I was so caught up in the yogic ideal that a person's value comes from inside, not outside, that I just assumed that yoga publications in the world would uphold that same ideal.

Wrong.

From the Mouths of Three-Year-Olds

Since 2002, I have been teaching yoga to people of all ages, infants through seniors. I've also seen the practice evolve (or devolve) with its explosive popularity from a practice based largely in awareness and mindfulness to one based largely in self-indulgence and aesthetics.

At its best, I've worked with rooms full of women of every shape, size, and background, who all walk out of a practice feeling beautiful. At its worst, I've worked with a 3-year-old girl (the child of two movie stars and already a pint-sized, lip-glossed bombshell) who in the middle of class, kept gravitating to the mirror and crying out loud, "I'm ugly! I'm so ugly!"

What's Society Got to Do with It?

One of the ultimate goals of yoga is to learn how to see beyond *maya*, illusion. The concept of *maya* is that our worlds are colored by our knowledge and experience, our prejudices and our biases. We see the world as we are trained to see to it, rather than how it really is. Put in the context of body image, *maya* would be body dysmorphia, seeing ourselves as "fat" or "ugly" as subjective indicators of our worth (or lack thereof).

When our body image filters are tinted with Photoshop, plastic surgery, and size 0 runway models, it becomes hard to just accept child-bearing hips, pancake chests, and the laugh lines that come naturally with age and, yes, smiling.

Sadly, these same judgments that adults place upon themselves are often projected onto their children. For the most part, the expectations are well intended. Everyone wants to see his or her child thrive and be accepted ... and pretty (read: thin) people are popular people. But all too often, these misguided intentions become hurtful and shameful. This can look like 5-year-olds being told they can't have cake at a party, 9-year-olds being put on diets, and teenagers being told they are fat in front of just about anyone within earshot.

So we wind up with a cadre of humiliated children with low self-esteem, convinced they are fat (read: ugly) and good for nothing. And the other kids aren't helping to ease this perception, either. Rampant name-calling, chiding, and bullying all contribute to children who hate their bodies ... and themselves. We need to move past this self-destructive spiral, to create self-worth in all children, to empower everyone to love him or herself.

We need yoga.

I wish I'd had it when I was a kid.

Mean Girls

Growing up in southern California, poor body image wasn't something you had to inflict on yourself. Your peers did that favor for you.

Personally, I stopped hanging out at the beach by tenth grade because I didn't like how I looked in a bikini. I wasn't what you would consider fat, mind you. In fact, I was the consummate athlete, working out (hard!) for hours every single day. But I wasn't what you would consider skinny, either. And the other girls were. Every day, I would spend hours trying to tie a sweatshirt around my waist *just so*, at just the right height, just the right angle, in an attempt to visually trim my waist. My boyfriend wasn't allowed to touch my stomach.

And then, finally, in my freshman year of college, I decided to limit myself to one small bowl of granola and one small bowl of vegetables, plus at least two forms of exercise a day. Even still, all I could see was fat. Fat, fat, fat, fat, fat.

Man, did I need yoga.

Woman in the Mirror

As an adult who discovered yoga for the first time at age 30, it was the first time in my life that I was told that it is okay to fall. That's right. It's okay to fall. This was a huge revelation, especially to someone who had been told her whole life that she needed to be perfect. How empowering to learn that the best I can do is the best that can be expected of me! And, what's more, to realize that at any given moment I am always giving the most I have to give.

Growing up, I truly believed that I had to be the best at everything: the president of every group, the captain of every team. And I had one life goal and one life goal only. I was going to go to Stanford. For four years of high school, I was top of the class, top of the SATs, top of the teams, winning awards and honors, and generally believing I was invincible. Then came the dreaded thin envelope and my world came crashing down. I wasn't going to Stanford. I wasn't the Golden Child. As far as I was concerned, I wasn't worth the paper that @#%#% letter was written on.

For ten years—*ten years*—I beat myself up for being useless, worthless, after not getting into that school. That is, until I stepped into Bryan Kest's yoga class. I could have sworn he was talking *to me* when he said it was okay to fall. It was like living in that song "Killing Me Softly" ... how did he know me so well when we'd never met? How did he know what I needed to hear? (Or, perhaps, is it just what we all need to hear?)

When we learn to accept that we are perfect in and of ourselves, by default we also learn that everyone else is as well. Take it one step further: if I can accept the perfection of my current self, then I must, in turn, accept the body that contains me. The process of learning self-acceptance is a difficult one. We are taught from an early age to be both critical and humble—two sides, in a way, of the same coin and ourselves.

Paying It Backward and Forward

In yoga, there is a certain code of ethics—the *yamas* and *niyamas*—that leads us beyond this illusion and self-abuse. The first of the *yamas*, *ahimsa* or nonviolence, says that we must be kind to ourselves as we are kind to others. This is sort of the Golden Rule of yoga. It reminds us that at every moment of every day, we can be our own best friend or our own worst enemy. Ultimately, it comes down to our relationship with ourselves and our comfort within our own skin.

The reason I started mini yogis® yoga for kids was because I wanted to give children this gift that I didn't receive until I was 30. I couldn't stop thinking how my life might have been different had I been introduced to yoga at age 3 instead of 30, if I knew I could not fail.

When I work with kids now, I work hard to make sure that every child feels good about himself or herself and feels empowered. No matter what weight loss goals the children I work with might have, I make sure they understand the reason I am there is not to make them look prettier, thinner, or more perfect, but rather to help them see how perfect they already are.

Body Positivity without Pom-Poms

In my yoga classes with children, all of the focus is on effort and not on "right" and "wrong." A kid's yoga practice is likely the only arena in a child's life where competition and perfection don't come into play. Yoga acknowledges that all people are inherently perfect *within* their idiosyncrasies and imperfections. In fact, falling is a really great indication of effort … something to be applauded and celebrated, rather than condemned.

Of course, it's important—especially with pretcens and teens—that your students do not think you are pandering to them or patronizing them. It's not enough to just wait for a kid to tell you he's fat and then react with "No, you're not." It's important to know which kids have low self-esteem and make sure you are *proactive* in reinforcing positive thought … before the negative thought even appears.

When I have kids with low self-esteem or poor body image, we will work on mantras, repeating a positive affirmation over and over in our heads to the exclusion of other thoughts. And if a student says anything negative about herself, we quickly work to change the thought and change the words.

When a teenager with poor body image walks into class, tugging down on her shirt or failing to take off his bulky sweatshirt, I comment on how good they look that day and *instantly* their energy shifts, because I say it like I mean it (and I do!), not like a well-trained seal who always reflexively responds "You're not ugly."

What Do Boys and Girls Have in Common?

Of course, these issues aren't limited to teens and 'tweens. Body image awareness starts at a very early age. According to Britain's *Daily Mail*, the number of children under age 10 being treated for anorexia doubled in 2011 over the 2010 figures, with girls *as young as 5 years old* being treated for severe cases. They also estimate that 25 percent of all girls 10 years old are on a self-imposed weight loss diet.[1]

In my personal experience, perhaps the most disconcerting trend in body image awareness is the growing number of boys who are becoming obsessed with their weight and bodies. While our awareness of this issue has been largely focused on girls, I am meeting more and more boys with the same issues.

I have one particular boy I've worked with for years. He carried his baby fat perhaps a bit longer than some others, but he never looked overweight or out of shape. I spent a lot of time helping him boost his self-esteem and telling him how fabulous he was (not just on the outside, but particularly on the inside), and while he was in my classes, it seemed to work. He sat up taller, smiled more, and carried himself with pride. But the kids at school kept tearing him down, and every week we'd start over with me reminding him of how incredible he really was.

Then he went to New York to spend the summer with his (female) cousin, a club-hopping freshman at NYU. This 17-year-old boy came back at the end of summer a good 10 pounds leaner and clearly feeling great about himself. He even bragged to me about how much he ate that day. And it was *a lot*. This from the boy who was usually so embarrassed about his weight and his looks that eating for him was a shameful addiction and something he didn't want to talk about. And then as I came closer to him, I realized that he had just brushed his teeth. At four in the afternoon. I quickly discovered that he had just thrown up his meal, and I wanted to cry.

I'd never seen this boy happier than when he discovered bulimia.

And here's the challenge: if I continue to talk about how good he looks and bolster his self-esteem, he'll know his eating disorder is "working." And if I don't, he'll think it's not working and is likely to take it to even deeper extremes.

What would you do?

Sticks and Stones

The things that people say to us when we are very young—particularly the things that hurt the most—are the things that tend to stick. Beyond the poor body image that ridiculed children grow up with is the skewed body image they will carry with them their entire lives. It is not uncommon for someone who was teased as a kid to always carry that "fat kid" label with them throughout their adult lives...no matter how thin they get, or what measures they have to take to get there.

The beauty of yoga—particularly at an early age—is its nonjudgmental nature. Unlike other popular sports that revere the physical aesthetic, forcing children to diet (or even starve) and work through injuries, yoga encourages students to love who they are and be mindful of their injuries and/or limitations. That's not to say that yoga promotes complacency. It doesn't. But it does promote constant self-study and introspection (*svadhyaya*), so that you are living to your own ideal of the best you can be, instead of someone else's.

Of course, not all children have negative issues with body image. Some are quite proud and uninhibited about their bodies, regardless of shape and size. I have a girl I work with who is 8 and very tall and slender. She has a penchant for short-short shorts and small tops that show off her belly. Her 10-year-old sister likes to wear fake tattoos on her low back, just above the line of her miniskirts. And their mother is fine with it. As long as they feel good about themselves, they can wear what they want.

Now, I look back at pictures of my sister and me growing up in the 1970s and the outfits we used to wear. Funny, they aren't that much different from these girls' (minus the tattoos). But that was a different time. Back then, we were just kids who were hot from playing and wanted to cool off. These days, with the constant objectification and hypersexualization of women—and girls!—little girls can't wear skimpy outfits without men leering at them like predators.

On the flip side of the coin, I have another girl, age 3 and precious as can be, who is pretty well overweight for her age. But she couldn't care less. Let's call her Vivian. She loves to roll up her shirt, lift up her shirt, take off her shirt. Not the least bit self-conscious. Healthy.

She is in a class of five children, ages 3 and 4, and after meditation, they love to pile up on my lap one at a time into a lotus tower. One day, four kids were on the pile and Vivian starts bounding up—huge smile on her face—to be "the cherry on top." Suddenly another girl squealed "Not her! It will hurt!" And Vivian deflated like a popped balloon.

I don't know how to explain it, but I could tell that Vivian knew the girl didn't mean *one more person* would hurt (we do five every time). It meant that Vivian would hurt them. And instead Vivian was the one who wound up hurt.

I quickly put out the fire by taking everyone off the tower and offering Vivian the highly coveted space directly on my lap. Then I talked to the kids about everyone getting a turn and that I will never, ever do anything with them that will hurt them, and about being nice. To everyone. Always.

My Little Belly

I also work extensively with adults and have a well-viewed YOGAthletica channel on YouTube. A few months ago someone posted the comment "I love your little belly" on my most popular video. And I was *mortified*. The whole world could see the comment and laugh.

Now, I don't know if the comment was meant as an actual compliment or a dig, but I went ahead and clicked "like." Not because I appreciated the comment or was happy about it, but because I was proud of myself for not deleting it.

For all the yoga and all the practice I do, day in and day out, I won't pretend that I wouldn't still like a flatter stomach, maybe some smaller hips. Heck, it would be great to lose just five pounds. Maybe ten. I wouldn't complain if it were fifteen … because I'm a yogini, but I'm still human. I try my best to accept my body, but through it all, I do always remember that it's what's inside that really counts.

And, quite frankly, I really like what I see.

1. Sophia Borland. "The Anorexia Victims Aged Five: Doctors Blame Ultra-Slim Celebrities as Almost 100 Under-9s Are Treated in Hospital." *Daily Mail*, www.dailymail.co.uk/news/article-2020765/Children-aged-FIVE-treated-anorexia-Doctors-blame-ultra-slim-celebrities.html (accessed March 2014).

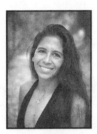 **Shana Meyerson** founded mini yogis® yoga for kids in March 2002. A pioneer in the children's yoga community, Shana has taught teachers all over the world how to teach children in a fun, safe, and mindful way. Her intuitive and integrative approach to teaching allows her to positively change the lives of both typically developing and special needs children. Trained in classical yoga by one of the world's most renowned yogis, Sri Dharma Mittra, Shana considers her teaching an offering to the sweet innocence of children and the lives that lay ahead of them. www.miniyogis.com

Author photo by Madoka Hamlin.

PART FIVE

Gender and Sexuality

This section asks us to consider how yoga shows up for people of different gender identities and sexual orientations. With that lens, the authors take us through a conversation about how yoga and body image is far from a conversation limited to women (as it is often seen), but rather is part of a much broader consideration for all of us.

Rosie Molinary starts us off with her personal story of the various ways she felt alienated from her body—particularly in how men viewed and treated her body over the years. She shares how yoga, quite unexpectedly, became a way for her to claim her body as her own with love.

Next, Dr. Kerrie Kauer weaves us through her experience as an athlete, particularly once she came out. Using that as a springboard, she also shares her research on athleticism and sexuality and how they intersect at the body—and what yoga can do to help integrate how we all feel about our bodies.

Then Bryan Kest takes us into his experiences of masculinity, growing up emulating his tough father, and how yoga gave him a way to redefine both masculinity and his relationship with his own body.

Next, Ryan McGraw ends the book with his experience as a male yogi with cerebral palsy. After first assuming that yoga wasn't for him, and hoping that his friends wouldn't find out he was practicing because it didn't fit their ideas about what it means to be a man, he found his way both on and off the mat through yoga—and in so doing, inspires us to do the same.

Finally, Dr. Audrey Bilger shares her experience of alienation as the only visible, out lesbian on a college campus, an ensuing encounter with a hostile environment, and how yoga helped her navigate it all and come back to her body.

MEETING MY OWN BODY

Rosie Molinary

"My uncle says Puerto Rican girls are F-I-N-E FINE," he hisses, his hands groping for me in the crowd getting on the bus after school. He is in third grade; I am in fourth grade. Already I have grown ashamed of my body, of my looks, of who I am supposed to be because (as I see it) I speak Spanish.

This is what happens every day after school. A band of boys who have decided I am a target because of my Puerto Ricanness swarm at the bus door when I try to get on it, sticking their hands out, trying desperately to cop a feel of my nonexistent bottom.

I swat their hands away. I cover my body. I say no. It doesn't get better.

Checking Out

When I finally get on that dark tin cylinder, I look for a window seat on the other side of the bus, so they can't see me. Finally, I just start missing the bus after school. A teacher sees me and loads me in his car and drives me home. Though I don't tell him what's going on, I keep missing the bus or finding reasons to stay after school because it is the only way I know that I can keep myself safe.

213

Soon enough, I will find another way to keep myself safe. I will disassociate from my body. I will bind it, cover it, ignore it. I will pretend it doesn't exist. I will not derive pleasure from it. I will unknow it, because what I am learning from the boys around me is that my body is different and, if unleashed, could be dangerous to me. It could put me in harm's way.

I am so scared of getting any attention for my body that I pull away from it. I fill my brain with as much smarts as I can fit in there. I do as much good as I can. I become the living embodiment of the good girl, because my body, I understand, could be very bad and something must make up for it.

Still, there are moments where my body startles me. On the day of my high school graduation, I put on a dress my mother has sewn for me. It is a white high halter dress that falls to my ankles, modestly showing just my shoulders and neck. Days earlier, a friend chopped off my long curls. My hair falls in a short, bouncy bob. In the mirror, I don't recognize myself, but I willingly smile at that girl. I imagine she is different from me, and she will be the one leaving for North Carolina to start a new life in college. I startle myself when I realize that I like how she looks. Up until now, I have mostly not even known how I looked.

That night, when a friend sees me, his eyes grow wide. "You look slutty," he tells me. There is music playing and I cannot make out my friend's words over the bass. For a second, I think he has told me I look pretty. A woozy kind of proud embarrassment passes over my face. It is one of the few times I have thought about my body, much less felt proud of it.

"What?" I scream in his ear, because this is the kind of compliment I want to be sure I hear. I want to know if he sees the girl I saw in the mirror when I was getting ready. I want to know if she is who I am becoming.

"YOU LOOK SLUTTY," he says louder, disapproving.

The proud embarrassment turns to two parts of shame: shame for looking slutty, shame for being proud of my body and looks for a second.

The Body as Shared Reality

Even though I ignore my body, it keeps developing. I have breasts I want no one to notice, a curvy figure that mortifies me. I let my tumbling curls hide my face, hide me. Where I live at the time, mine is a body type few people have. I try to believe that I don't have it either.

In my 20s, the experience of a potent new crush is debilitating because I am petrified by what I feel. When a fondness for a friend turns into something more, I try to talk myself out of it, acutely aware that falling for him would mean I could no longer live in my disassociated world. One night, we find ourselves together in the midst of a volatile situation. As a good girl, I know how to smooth most everything over. When the crisis passes and it is just me and my crush left to talk about it, he moves to me, and I look at him, shyly. My eyes track over his strong face, all angles and searing green eyes, memorizing it.

"You did great." He slips his fingers under my chin, tilting it toward him. I close my eyes and then reopen them to find him pressing toward me, surprising me with one of our many kisses I will replay for years.

"Go out with me," he pleads. I want nothing more than to do this, for it all to be this easy, to be the type of woman who can hop into his gunmetal-gray jeep and look out over the city with him, his hand casually draped over my thigh, as we move from bar to club, from screaming at a football game on the television to dancing unself-consciously to Eminem on a crowded dance floor, pushed up against him, breathing each other's air. But it terrifies me too, the list of possibilities such a decision would create.

"I can't," I whisper, placing my hand on his arm and then slowly backing away. My fingers touch the inside of his forearm for as long as I can before the distance becomes too much.

Over the years, I battle this intense attraction. I am terrified of my feelings for him, overwhelmed by how much there is to lose, so I play it as safe as I can. We kiss, and I walk away. He shares intimate details of his life that he has never told anyone. I do not match his candor. He senses my withholding, and confronts me. "Why are you so damned closed?" he asks one Saturday afternoon.

I can't answer him, so I do what I have learned how to do when things get hard: I leave. The distance I create is our living metaphor. As I drive away from him, tears stinging my eyes over the truth that creating this space is both the last thing I want to be doing and the most important thing I can do, I am overwhelmed with questions. If I really share my heart with him, will I lose it? And how could I ever let him get to know my body when I am scared of it, ashamed of it, do not even know it myself? Could I be good enough to have him forever? Is it even "good enough" that I have to be, or is it "true enough"? And if it is true enough, how can I be true to someone else—to his soul and his body—when I have not even learned to be true to myself?

Over time, I confirm that what is essential about me—what he loves about me—does not come from my body. What is essential about me is the way I work ceaselessly for my passions, the way I feel and live my compassion, how I embrace my history and heritage, my self-sufficiency and independence, my surprising edge and developing confidence. But while I am not my body, I begin to understand that my body is my vehicle, my system for enjoying and experiencing life. Really inhabiting the body is a shared personal reality; it is both expression and sensation. I have not yet synthesized this lesson. I know I want to be the embodiment of this way of being, and so I start hungering for how it might come to me, how I might come to it. I do not yet know how to feed the hunger.

Inviting the Sensation

More years pass by me. I explore love and run from it for many of the same reasons. As an impassioned high school teacher, I live out my disassociation with my body in whole new ways. I work too hard and too long. I don't feed myself well. Life keeps handing you the lesson you need to learn until you learn it, my later self will come to understand, but I am not there yet so I keep giving and not replenishing, keep acting as if I don't have time to care for my body when actually the opposite is true.

Eventually, it catches up to me. My body gives out, and I yield to an epic sickness that forces me to sit at home for weeks in order to heal and recover.

I realize I do not know how to teach in a different way, that teaching high school is my addiction, and I figure out that I have to do something different professionally if I am to physically make it. Running away is still the only real tool I have in my toolbox when things get hard.

I start over from what feels like rock bottom. I leave the career I thought I would have until I retired. I start a master's degree program in Fine Arts that forces me, finally, to claim my voice. And I find yoga, which leads me, finally, to settle into my body.

Something Greater

Yoga comes to me in an e-mail. The college where I work as an administrator is offering a weekly lunchtime yoga class. Because I am still prone to work rather than taking that lunch break, there is a knowing that comes over me when I first read the e-mail.

I need this, I tell myself with an absoluteness that startles me. Consciously, I cannot figure out why it is I need yoga, but subconsciously it feels like the truth. I am not sure if I think my hips need it or my heart, but even though I know nothing about yoga, even though I don't know anyone who practices it, I need to do it. I sign up before I can convince myself that I need that hour to work more.

I show up for my first yoga class in soccer shorts and a concert T-shirt. I grab a spot where the sunshine bounces into the conference room and sit on my teal mat, smiling greetings to each person who enters, anticipating the class. I have no idea what is to come, how by just trying not to work one hour where I would normally have squeezed as much productivity out of myself as I could, I might be led to something else entirely, something greater than just a little break once a week.

As I piece together my practice, week after week, I become more confident of the flow and poses. I close my eyes. I breathe. I don't care if I am good at any of it because whatever I am doing, however I am doing it, feels good and that is enough. I don't even have to be the good girl and follow every single instruction or suggestion the teacher gives. I take the modifications. I breathe when it feels right to me. I don't make myself work so hard if all I want to do it is rest in child's pose. I close my eyes for the entire practice and forget anyone else is there. On that mat, every single Wednesday, it is just me and a gentle, guiding voice. I am in charge of my body and what it is feeling, and what I realize is that as it releases something physical, I release something emotional too.

I am in charge of me, I come to understand as I forward fold and Warrior and backbend. And my body and what it feels is not something I should fear. If I don't like something, I don't have to do it, but I don't have to hide in order to not do it. I can just decide no or yes at any given moment. My body is not separate from me, nor is it me. It is the vessel that I have been given to experience this life, and I have been denying myself part of its expression.

A Whole out of Parts

As I become less afraid of physically feeling my body, as I come to understand that feeling my body will not slay me, I find myself wishing for one pose every class. Please lead us to Pigeon, I silently chant every class. And when she does, I settle into it not with the ease of the bendy back poses that are like second nature for me but with an internal scream. What I understand as I fold over my shin is that what I am asking for with Pigeon, what I am eager for, is feeling my body. After a lifetime of desperately trying to feel nothing in my body, I am begging for the most physically sensational pose to make up for lost time, to awaken my knowing.

Emotions flood me and tears rush to my eyes as I hold the pose. I think of darting, like I always have. And yet, what I realize as I breathe in and out, and release more deeply into the sensation, is there is nothing I need more at this moment than this pose. Moreover, I cannot just power my way through. I have to be in this pose to transcend it; I cannot run away to escape it; I have to breathe into it. I have to experience what my body feels and needs and has to say. For the first time, really.

When I do that, everything changes just a little bit, and when I string together practices like that, days like that, the whole landscape changes, the continent shifts. My walls tumble, my boundaries shift. I am no longer bound by how my body—or someone else's experience of my body—might betray me. I am informed by how my soul can take care of my body and my body can do the same for my soul. I am a collaborating force, emboldened by both sensation and expression.

That is the gift of yoga. It teaches you what you most need to know. For me, it is about making a whole out of parts that I thought could exist separately. Yoga heals what is most broken, tends what most needs tending, leads you to forgive what most needs grace, and encourages you to face what most needs consideration. The mat becomes a personal laboratory, the poses your proof.

Soon, the weekly yoga class in the college's conference room is no longer enough. I sometimes close the door to my office and lead my body and soul to what it most needs from the mat. I find yoga classes outside of the workplace. I realize that I can give myself this gift any time. I do not have to wait for someone to lead me into my body. I can do that for myself.

Making the Connection

Once I have been physically emboldened, I find I am more personally possessed. I realize my body does not have to scare me, that no one will ever control my body but me, that the boys by the bus door are long gone from my life, and that, even if they weren't, I now have everything I need to chase them away. I do not have to run from anyone. I do not have to run from my body. But I can run. And I do. I cycle. I push up. I learn to swim. I surf. I dance. I paint. I write my truths. I let myself fall in ridiculous love, despite its inherent risk. I travel. I Namaste. I live with all of me.

Yoga helped your body image, someone might conclude and, absolutely, it has, but it is so much more than that. What yoga did was connect my whole body, helping me reimagine myself so that I was no longer the disparate parts of a body and a soul. Yoga served as a catalyst toward personal unity for me. It taught me to not be afraid of any sensation, that I could breathe through it all and get to the other side, that I have everything I need inside of me. I had never been afraid to do the mental and emotional work before but had always been afraid of feeling the sensation of anything. Yoga taught me that sometimes inviting the sensation is the best thing you can do for yourself. All you need to do is connect with your soul and breathe, because you already have everything you need deep within.

I file this little piece of information away: it will always be easy for me to disassociate from my body. When things get hard, I will choose my default, which is to go all cerebral and whole heart with no body awareness in sight. So I create a world that is sensitive to the fact that I have in me the ability to disassociate, and I do what I can to ground myself from it happening and to catch myself when it does. And because it took me so long to figure it out, to mend, to create a world where all of me can live, I do what I can to empower others to create a world where they can be their whole selves—so that we can all be ready for the love of our lives which, as it turns out, wasn't that crush from years ago, but me.

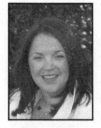

Rosie Molinary is an author and educator who empowers women to embrace their authentic selves so they can live their passion and purpose and give their gifts to the world. Rosie is the author of *Beautiful You: A Daily Guide to Radical Self-Acceptance* and *Hijas Americanas: Beauty, Body image, and Growing Up Latina*. Rosie teaches body image at the University of North Carolina at Charlotte, offers workshops and retreats for women, and speaks on self-acceptance, body image, media literacy, the Latina experience, and social justice around the country. www.rosiemolinary.com

Author photo by Deborah Triplett.

THE ATHLETIC YOGI: SEXUALITY AND IDENTITY THROUGH THE BODY

Dr. Kerrie Kauer

I am a Title IX baby. Title IX is a federal law that states *"No person in the United States shall, on the basis of sex, be excluded from participation in, be denied the benefits of, or be subjected to discrimination under any education program or activity receiving federal financial assistance."* [1] I was born in 1975, two years after its implementation, and growing up in Pittsburgh, I was exposed to many opportunities to engage in sports and organized athletics, as well as receive the principal benefit of Title IX for girls and women: equal opportunity in education. While many people assume Title IX is a law enacted for athletics, its initial purpose was educational reform to end sex discrimination, particularly in higher education, however, it applies to all education sectors that receive federal financial assistance.

I was incredibly active in my youth. I swam, ran track and field, played softball, volleyball, and basketball, and participated in every form of physical activity possible at recess. I loved the sense of pushing myself and trying new things—climbing trees, riding BMX trails with my older brother, roller and ice skating. I was strong, empowered, whole, and alive when I was engaged in any kind of competitive sport or physical activity. I felt free.

Freedom in the Body

During that period in my life, I rarely worried about my body shape or size, and I had a positive body image. Yet I was not immune to the conversations that ensued around me by teammates, parents, and coaches. One of my teammates and best friends at the time struggled with her body image and weight and regularly commented on my ability to "eat whatever I wanted" or wear a certain clothing size.

However, my mother would regularly make comments to me about my eating habits, warning me that someday I would have to change my diet because my body would change, and I would begin to gain weight. I usually heard this after I scarfed a sleeve or two of chocolate chip cookies after basketball practice. In her mind, she was looking out for me. The focus was never really on the healthiness of what I was eating, but the quantity in which I was indulging.

Like most adolescents, I began navigating my sexual identity early in high school and had my first love experience my freshman year with another girl. There was a great deal of shame and secrecy around my feelings, and I kept this part of my identity hidden until after graduating college. Being athletic felt more comfortable to me than hyperfeminine or traditional forms of girlhood and femininity. I didn't prefer dresses or frilly feminine clothes, so sports felt natural and helped me feel comfortable in my body. Paradoxically, I heard many discriminatory comments and disparaging homophobic remarks from people around me in sports, whether they were coaches, teammates, or even the sports media.

With messages like this and other heteronormative ideologies that US society perpetuated, I believed I needed to keep my sexuality a secret. These messages occurred and even intensified once I went off to college. Several of my coaches were lesbians, but a cloud of silence hovered over their sexuality, and there were always rumors and accusations floating around with younger or newer athletes on each of my teams. These silences around sexuality sent a very clear message to me that being a lesbian was something to be ashamed of and to hide. During the four years of my undergraduate degree, I didn't know a single "out" lesbian at my college, and I certainly wasn't brave enough to be the first.

It was during my undergraduate education that my body started changing and I began associating more negative feelings and emotions with my body than positive ones. Like many college students, I gained a significant amount of weight, though I was still very active playing college basketball. I also started drinking alcohol for the first time in my life, and my body reacted by losing and gaining weight consistently during season and in the off-season. Coaches throughout my career would regularly discuss the bodies of other athletes, saying things like, "So and so looks like she gained a third grader, she put on so much weight."

But my changing body wasn't only attributed to the cliché freshman fifteen. Because of all the weight training and physical conditioning, I could never fit quite right into dresses; my back was too broad and my shoulders a little too big. To this day, I still walk in heels like they are high-top basketball shoes. Most jeans wouldn't fit because my quads were more muscular than the inseam in any pants would allow, so I often opted for more loose-fitting men's jeans. After spending a lifetime as an athlete, during the middle of my senior season, I tore my anterior cruciate ligament (ACL) and needed reconstructive surgery. My identity as an athlete was shattered; I was depressed and not active and turned to food and alcohol to fill the hole in my soul.

The Athletic Aesthetic

It was also during this time that the "athletic aesthetic" became more of a norm—more so than the waif-like images that circulated the media in the early nineties. The mainstream beauty ideal began to shift at the same time I transitioned from playing basketball to becoming a college coach myself. I remember subscribing to Condé Nast's *Women's Sports & Fitness* magazine, a periodical that saw only four years of circulation.[2] Just one year earlier, the Women's Basketball National Association (WNBA) launched successfully, the US women's Olympic teams won an unprecedented amount of medals, and the image of the female athlete became more normalized. I clearly remember the desire to look as toned and muscular as the women in the magazines—and I remember feeling frustrated that I couldn't achieve that goal. The images in the magazine fit into what Pirkko Markula and colleagues described as "firm but shapely, fit but sexy, strong but thin," and as paradoxical as that was, I was determined to mold myself into this unrealistic ideal for *my* body.[3]

As many feminist scholars have argued, this new marketing of health and beauty fits into commodity feminism or the idea that the actions of the body are the center of liberation for women; in other words, you've made it as a woman when you can look like those images. Because the body is so wrapped up in the outward appearance of one's health, the body that doesn't look "healthy" (i.e., thin and toned) has been associated with individual and moral laxity. Spurred by consumer capitalism, this burgeoning athletic aesthetic works to sell products in the marketplace (e.g., fitness memberships, Botox, lap-band surgery, pharmaceuticals) while simultaneously creating unrealistic images for most women in North America. Women athletes who appear too muscular or strong are labeled masculine and lesbian, or somehow as failed women.

As this image has shifted over time, the female athletic body has been slightly more acceptable as long as it's within the normative boundaries of muscularity. Male athletes rarely have to contend with paradoxical norms around masculine bodies. Part of what is defined as masculinity in Western culture is athleticism, and while some sports are deemed more feminine (e.g., gymnastics, figure skating), male bodies in these spaces still require strength and muscularity that mark them as masculine in the public sphere. Women athletes who face this paradox have also gone to great lengths to perform their gender appropriately within societal expectations. What this means is often complying with media desires to portray an ultra-feminine, "heterosexy" image, and the plethora of provocative, seminude, and nude images of female athletes has hit an all-time high.

As a college professor, one assignment I have my students do is Google the words "female athlete" and this point becomes shockingly clear. It is particularly interesting to note that the most successful female athletes in terms of their athletic prowess and success (i.e., winning) are often invisible, while less successful but more beauty-conforming female athletes receive more endorsements, magazine covers, and television commercials. Tennis player Anna Kournikova is the best example in modern sports history of a female athlete who never won a singles tournament, yet received more press and endorsements than any other athlete during that era based solely on her physical appearance.

Sports and Safety

As a young coach, I consumed this ideal and soon became obsessed with my workout schedule, followed the routines laid out in magazines, and began dieting. I fell into the spectrum of disordered eating on the end of the continuum that wouldn't be categorized as a clinical eating disorder, but *disordered eating and disordered body image*—an issue that faces a significant amount of women in the United States. Disordered eating (as well as clinical eating disorders) also includes a host of behaviors related to exercise addiction or over-exercising. Now, after years of reflection, it isn't surprising to me that my struggles with my body occurred at the same time I came out to my family and friends as a lesbian, and my insecurity about my worth in the world became entangled in the outward appearance of my body.

This period in my life was riddled with contradictions and confusion. On the one hand, sports felt like an outlet for me or a safe space to be around teammates and like-minded women. My personal experience during these formative years led me to believe that lesbian women were more comfortable in their bodies. What I loved (and love) about the lesbian community that I was newly discovering was that there was so much body diversity and gender performance in the communities with whom I associated that mainstream images were rarely a point of discussion. Yet research about lesbians and body image both supports and refutes my experiences. According to some studies, lesbians have less concern with physical appearance, internalize the norm of thinness less from the media, are less involved with maintaining an ideal appearance, and are less likely to use exercise to control weight.[4]

However, some feminist scholars have argued that lesbians may not differ from heterosexual women in body dissatisfaction or eating disorders/disordered eating because lesbians have experienced the same gender socialization while growing up and thus are pressured to achieve the same culturally ideal body as heterosexual women. In other words, one's gender is more significant to their relationship with their bodies than their sexual identity. To this end, research has shown that lesbians and heterosexual women are similar in terms of pursuit of thinness,[5] behaviors related to bulimia,[6] and body dissatisfaction.[7][8] What I would argue is important about this research and my own experiences is that essentializing groups, whether it's "all women" or "all lesbians," is problematic, but society, as well as the yoga community, does it all the time. More on this a bit later.

The Professional Body

I coached women's basketball for three years before heading off to graduate school to get a master's degree in sport psychology. Looking back, part of what I was interested in doing was helping young female athletes feel okay in their bodies and about their sexual identity, probably because I needed the help and healing myself. I began reading about other women's experience in sports and how homophobia affected them. I also began studying the body in more critical ways and how bodies have become socially constructed, the ways in which sexuality, gender, race, and social class help define the body. (And more recently, taking my research to explore the connections between the body, social justice, and anti-oppression work with yoga.)

Two years after finishing my doctoral program, I moved to southern California to take a tenure-track position in academia. I was still highly active and enjoyed running an average of four to five miles a day. After years of running, I found myself with osteoarthritis, a common problem associated with ACL reconstruction surgery, due to the wear and tear on my knee. My knee became so painful I couldn't get through a lecture standing, and my most comforting form of exercise, running, was slowly fading from my daily routine. A friend suggested Bikram yoga, and after my first class I was hooked. After three weeks I was off the anti-inflammatory drugs for my knee and started to gain great mobility in my knees, ankles, and hips.

Yoga and Coming Home to the Body

Like many Westerners who are introduced to yoga, I went to heal an injury and discovered the many benefits that yoga provided for my mind, body, and spirit. Bikram was the perfect entry point for me because it felt challenging and lacked the "fluff" I had typically associated with yoga; it provided me with some of the structure and militarism that felt so familiar from my sports experience. Several years into my Bikram practice I started branching out to find other practices and regularly took up Ashtanga and vinyasa flow classes soon after I did my first leadership intensive with Off the Mat, Into the World, an organization that connects grassroots activism to the yoga community.

One of the most profound effects of my practice is with my relationship to myself and my body. I am gentler with myself, for the most part. As a woman in this society, even with all my feminist politics, I am still not immune to the inundation of messages about beauty, thinness, and the unrealistic expectations this culture has for my body shape and size. And many of the images that are distributed by the marketing and advertising of yoga fit neatly into the health/fitness/body industrial complex that perpetuates the same images I saw in that Condé Nast magazine.

While I loved the practice of Bikram yoga and the healing benefits I received, I grew tired of the constant remarks about reshaping bodies, weight loss, and fitting into tiny Shakti yoga shorts. I felt frustrated at the constant gender emphasis on how bodies moved. Men's bodies were "less flexible because of their muscular strength." Teachers often perpetuated the stereotypes that delineate women as weaker, petite, and demur, and generalized all men as strong and more muscular. When I'm doing particular postures that are challenging because I have tight shoulders from years of lifting weights, I don't want to hear that only men struggle with this issue. I grew increasingly frustrated with the essentializing gendered norms that were thrown about in those classes and eventually stopped going to Bikram yoga.

While other forms of yoga are not perfect with regard to gender-neutral language nor do many take on queer perspectives around sexuality, I found several studios that did not perpetuate body shame or hatred. I felt safe in other forms of yoga—embraced, in fact. My body has held on to a lot of the homophobia and shame from hiding my identity while I was younger, particularly as an athlete. My body remembered my 14-year-old self hiding and sneaking to call my girlfriend. My body remembered my 19-year-old self, feeling confused and scared when all I wanted to do was cry to my mom, but I was too afraid of disappointing her. While I had the intellectual tools through my graduate work and professional life, it has been through yoga that I feel like I have been able to disentangle many of the cultural messages I have received about my sexual identity, and that has led to more freedom and love of myself.

Appreciation

This is not a linear process, nor do I believe I have "arrived" somewhere in this journey. Just as with most things, my relationship with my body is in a constant negotiation, and while this dialogue has changed slightly throughout my life as an athlete and now a yogi, it remains a paradoxical experience. From the time I was in graduate school in kinesiology until my current tenure-track position, I have been surrounded by people interested in fitness, athletic bodies, body shaping and toning, and burning calories. Even when in specific feminist groups, I learned that many of us in this discipline struggled with our own body image, ranging from disordered body images to clinical eating disorders.

My experience in a kinesiology department put a constant focus on my own body and the expectation that my body should look a particular way. I've seen much discrimination from faculty in kinesiology departments because of the body shape of a graduate student or other faculty members, including in hiring practices! In the classroom I also felt hyper-aware of my own body. Was I thin and fit enough for aspiring students in exercise physiology or sport psychology to think I'm qualified to teach them? Research shows that women in academics are not taken as seriously, and fat women in particular are taken even less seriously, so I knew what I was feeling intuitively was well founded.

As a child, my sport experience felt embodied. Somewhere along the way, though, a schism occurred and instead of feeling fully integrated, I adopted more of a mechanistic outlook on my body. Yoga has brought me back to truth. The discourse in yoga has been the opposite, where my teacher is constantly reminding me that yoga is a journey and it might take several lifetimes to complete a posture—and that the most important thing is the breath. That mentality and philosophy help ground me and lessen the amount of body shaming I do to myself. In some of my classes where there are mirrors, which are typically associated with body objectification, I learn to love my body and appreciate holding a standing balancing posture or at least my ability to smile at myself when I fall out. And while I know that yoga has been saturated by the same commercialism and commodity feminism as other capitalist endeavors here in the West, I have hope that maybe it can lead to more body acceptance and love for more girls and women. While not all intention in yoga is about liberation from the hierarchal confines of consumer capitalism and the love of ones body *as it is*, I know from my experience that with the right instructor, intention, and shifting mentality of the body, yoga can become a tool to dismantle these systems.

1. R. Acosta and L. Carpenter. "Women in Intercollegiate Sport: A Longitudinal Study Twenty-Three Year Update, 1977–2000." *Women in Sport and Physical Activity Journal* (2000), 141–144.

2. "Condé Nast Set to Close Down a Magazine." *New York Times*, www.nytimes.com/2000/06/28/business/conde-nast-set-to-close-down-a-magazine.html (accessed March 2014).

3. P. Markula, A. Yiannakis, and M. Melnick. "Firm but Shapely, Fit but Sexy, Strong but Thin: The Postmodern Aerobicizing Female Bodies." *Contemporary Issues in Sociology of Sport* (2001), 237–258.

4. S. M. Strong, D. A. Williamson, R. G. Netemeyer, and J. H. Geer. "Eating Disorder Symptoms and Concerns About Body Differ as a Function of Gender and Sexual Orientation." *Journal of Social and Clinical Psychology*, 19 (2000), 240–255.

5. P. Wagenbach. "Lesbian Body Image and Eating Issues." *Journal of Psychology and Human Sexuality*, 15 (2003), 205–227.

6. K. Heffernan. "Eating Disorders and Weight Concern Among Lesbians." *International Journal of Eating Disorders*, 19 (1996), 127–138.

7. F. Moore and P. K. Keel. "Influence of Sexual Orientation and Age on Disordered Eating Attitudes and Behaviors in Women." *International Journal of Eating Disorders*, 34 (2003), 370–374.

8. A. K. Yancey, S. D. Cochran, H. L. Corliss, and V. M. Mays. "Correlates of Overweight and Obesity Among Lesbian and Bisexual Women." *Preventive Medicine*, 36 (2003) 676–683.

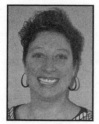 **Dr. Kerrie Kauer** is an associate professor of kinesiology at California State University, Long Beach. She has been an advocate for girls and women in sports and incorporates a feminist, social justice philosophy in her classroom and activism. Her research has examined social and psychological aspects of health, self-esteem, body image, and homophobia as it relates to girls and women in sports and physical activity. She has collaborated with Off the Mat, Into the World's Global Seva Challenge to raise awareness and resources for survivors of sex trafficking, and completed her 200-hour RYT training with Cloud Nine Yoga in 2012.

Author photo by Lauren Rauscher.

LIKE FATHER, LIKE SON

Bryan Kest

I wanted to be a stud. You know, a big, tall, ripped dude who could kick some major ass. As a young boy, a body that was six-foot-three with 220 pounds of muscle mass represented my ideal image of masculinity. And that was the image my buddies and I went for when we hit the gym. Not only was a man supposed to be buff and strong, but a "real man" had to be capable of fighting. In fact, I thought if a man couldn't physically intimidate and dominate another man, he wasn't a real man. Guys such as Sylvester Stallone, Dolph Lundgren, Clint Eastwood, and Arnold Schwarzenegger were the epitome of this ideal.

But I was exposed to violent masculinity before guys such as Arnold and Sylvester appeared on the big screen. I was like any other boy growing up in the suburbs of Detroit, or anywhere else in the United States, watching buffed-up superheroes like *The Incredible Hulk* on Saturday morning cartoons. Detroit, a hardscrabble, blue-collar town, wasn't unique in proliferating these images and attitudes for boys and men. What boy doesn't want to be the brave hero? It's what we've been told we should want, passed down through generations of men.

Starting at Home

In fact, my first influence on my idea of a "real man" came even earlier than my favorite cartoons. My biggest icon was my father, and he bought into all the trappings of masculinity. He was six-foot-one, big, strong, and aggressive. He kept a set of weights in our basement and owned a gun. He was not only the first but the biggest influence on me, and his version of masculinity was supported by everything I saw in the media (which surely influenced him too) and impacted the other images I gravitated toward later.

My dad dominated all the time. I saw him get into several fistfights on the streets. If someone cut him off while he was driving, he'd floor it and then they'd both jump out and go at it at a red light. I saw one guy come at my dad with a baseball bat, running straight toward our car. I was sitting in the back seat, scared shitless.

I remember being 8 years old, living in Detroit, and one of our neighbors screaming, "There's a burglar in the house! There's a burglar in the house!" I can still see my dad breaking out his gun and running down to her house with me following him. He wasn't jumping off buildings and didn't have wings sprouting off his back, but to the degree you could be an action hero and human, he was.

My dad embedded violence and aggressiveness in me—and then he left. I was 10 and there was nobody to control us. My brothers and I had been scared to death of him, but we weren't scared of my mom. He left and all hell broke loose at home. I was angry and there was no stopping me. But I wasn't unusual. I was just a boy who was strong enough and aggressive enough to fulfill this cultural image of masculinity.

Adrift

There was tons of testosterone in that house even after my dad left. I was one in a pack of four rowdy brothers who fed off each other. We fought and wrestled nonstop. My mom had two homes outside of our house: the principal's office and the emergency room. We even had our own seat in the emergency room.

I flunked fifth grade because I didn't apply myself. I wasn't doing my homework or even thinking about my grades. Because I flunked and because I needed discipline my mom couldn't give me, she sent me to a Catholic boarding military school where I was exposed to even more violence. They beat me the entire year that I lived there. They each had their weapon of choice, whether it was a hockey stick or a paddle. All the punishments were physical and I cried every weekend when I got to go home. I'd plead with my mom not to send me back. So after the year was up, I went back to public school. But that didn't last long.

I did what I wanted, instead of what I was supposed to do. By sixth grade, I was smoking dope and didn't care about school. By seventh grade, I was smoking in the bathroom, skipping school when I had the chance, and not doing any work. I'm not sure how I made it to ninth grade, but that was the last year of school in my life.

I promised my mom I'd go back, but I never did. I was working, into drugs, and getting in trouble. I went to court a lot and was put on probation as a juvenile. Surprisingly, I managed to avoid detention centers. But when I was in my 20s, I made it to jail a few times, whether it was a holding cell or a short sentence. I didn't even mind going to jail—I saw it as a place where tough guys ended up and it sounded good that I went. It was part of the street cred. Plus, I didn't have much to live for that made jail seem bad.

From Machismo to Yoga

Not only had my dad fit the bill in terms of masculinity, he'd achieved the American dream. He was a successful doctor and he had a beautiful wife, four beautiful kids, and a big house in the suburbs. And he was still fucking miserable. The American dream hadn't delivered.

He had a nervous breakdown and it started him searching. He would drag me to these churches where they were singing gospel. He was looking for Jesus or something, anything. But that didn't give him what he was looking for, so he would try something else.

Eventually, my dad retired at age 42 and moved to Hawaii without us. This was crazy—we were an American Jewish family. You didn't throw it all away to make a choice like this. You go to school, become a doctor, and be a good boy. Instead, he divorces his wife, leaves their four babies, and moves to the jungle. It's the most horrific story we could imagine to have in our family. But he fell in love with Hawaii and it removed him from the society we live in and its endless pressures.

And in Hawaii he discovered yoga. He started because he had a bad back and someone told him yoga would help. So he tried it and liked its effects, especially what it did to him mentally. He was a pressure cooker. Back in Detroit, he couldn't even make it to work without something outrageous happening because he was so aggressive. Between yoga and living among all the hippies from the sixties who had moved to Maui, he was less likely to blow his cap. He felt more relaxed and peaceful there, and the yoga released the tension in his body and mind.

He knew yoga was the best thing for his kids, but he knew we'd never do it if he asked us to. So he forced me to do it after my mom called and said, "You need to take him." My dad showed up and asked if I wanted to live with him in Hawaii. I did, and it gave him the opportunity to lay down his one house rule: "Do yoga every day or move the fuck out of my house."

Karma

My dad introduced me to David Williams, the Western pioneer of Ashtanga yoga, whom he had been working with for a month or two. I went with him every day, and I hated it. Weightlifting in the pursuit of the ideal masculine physique had made me stiff. I avoided stretching because it was too painful and my ego couldn't see any benefits. What was flexibility going to give me? It wasn't giving me anything that I thought was important. I hated yoga, but after six months of doing it, I couldn't deny how I felt—and I felt amazing. Plus, it was such a vigorous form of yoga that it maintained my muscle mass, which made it ego-gratifying as well.

It was undeniable—this was the path I needed to take. This is the path I knew I needed to take. My other teacher, Brad Ramsey, was espousing the spiritual teachings of yoga and made them important to me in addition to the physical practice. I was an aggressive kid, but I wasn't a stupid kid, and he inspired me to investigate yoga further. It was hard to deny its practicality and rationality. It just made sense to me.

The yogic teachings helped me realize the fallibility of that "tough guy" persona by exposing its true weaknesses. Those teachings led me to let go of my desire to get approval from others, mostly the people I found interesting and fun to hang out with. After all, I didn't want to hang out with a bunch of fucking sissies. I wanted to hang out with the tough, active, adrenaline-junkie kids who wanted to jump off cliffs.

That awareness started my inner battle with the angel and the devil. The angel would point out that these guys were not the best crowd to hang with. They were macho, aggressive, and even superficial. But I was torn because they were doing the fun things. I wanted to surf and woo women, and I didn't mind getting into a tussle along the way. The fun guys were just like that, but I realized the weakness in their mindset. I fought that battle for a long time by living in both worlds. I would sing "Hare Krishna" with my yoga teacher and then I would go hang out with the tough guys. I was living a double life.

A turning point came one day when I was walking down the street in Hawaii. As a white guy from the mainland living among the locals, I'd often get the "stink eye" and, if you made eye contact, a fight broke out. That happened to me all the time, but I wasn't going to back down. If you look at me, I'm going to look at you. But I remember the day I decided not to do that anymore. It may have seemed submissive or weak, but I decided to look away when people made eye contact. I made the conscious decision not to go down that road anymore.

The Big Shift

Even after that decision, though, my dual life continued for years, especially after I moved back to Detroit. I had lived with my dad in Hawaii for a year, but how many cliffs can you dive off? It got boring and I came to Michigan and started hanging with my old buddies only to return to the same dangerous and, often, illegal, pursuits as before—only taking it further and further. I may have learned yoga, but I wasn't practicing regularly. I was shopping for organic food during the day and fighting and smoking with my friends at night.

But after two particularly bad incidents and a drug bust, I withdrew from the world. I devoted the next few years of my life to my own transformation. I focused on my health, enrolled in college and started taking nutrition classes, and began a regimen of yoga in the morning, weights in the afternoon, and jumping rope at night. I was making a change and I was completely alone. It was a transition period, a withdrawal from an addiction. Through my new interests, I met new people. Whether it was through my macrobiotics seminar or my fitness classes, I was developing a new community, drawing to me people who were like the new me.

Although my anger and aggression didn't just evaporate, that mentality was steadily decreasing for me. In my life, power had always been about dominance and aggression. But now I understood real power exists in another way, in Jesus's example and the teachings of yoga. That other mentality can never win. It's impossible. That mentality will keep you in jail, and jail isn't winning. How can you be fulfilled in jail?

Beginning to Teach

A friend of mine moved to Pacific Palisades, California, and hired me to drive her car out. I thought Los Angeles was the best thing since sliced bread, and I thought "Man, I gotta live out here." So at 20, I moved West. I landed in Inglewood and lived in my car at the park for a few months. I'd get up in the morning, get ready at a health club affiliated to the one I belonged to in Detroit, and then I was off to work in a variety of restaurants around town. During that first year, I was not only busing tables and cutting sandwiches, but I was also a physical fitness trainer and, unbeknownst to my clients, I'd throw some yoga into all their sessions. I also started sharing the practice with my coworkers who were curious about this yoga thing. Eventually, I started teaching fitness and yoga in a few local gyms and had more and more private clients. I'd get on my motorcycle, drive to Malibu, and go from mansion to mansion, training and teaching yoga to private clients. And as time went on, I was invited to teach yoga at a center for eating disorders and got hired by the Center for Yoga. Teaching yoga became a full-time job at a time when there were very few studios in LA County and very few teachers.

Even though I was teaching, I was still caught up with my image and ego. But I walked my walk and worked on my stuff. And the things I emphasized then and continue to emphasize now are the issues I was facing. I was working out the things I had directly experienced—such as my anger, violence, vanity, and ego—as I taught, and I noticed people resonated with it. It was clear I wasn't the only one dealing with the problem of dealing with disappointment and the stress of not meeting one-dimensional cultural expectations.

What I taught then and continue to teach is how to use the practice, a step-by-step way to combat all those toxic images and get them out of my head. Yoga gives you the tools to make tangible changes. But the real yoga is not the physical postures. It's awareness and the state of mind you cultivate as you move through the *asanas*. Without that meditative quality, the postures aren't yoga and they're not healing. In fact, some use the physical practice to hang on to youth or gratify their ego in a number of ways, thereby exacerbating the issues that hurt us the most. I always say, "If you bring your shit into yoga, you turn your yoga into shit."

With awareness, a physical yoga practice becomes a tool to investigate your body. You have the opportunity to notice. There's almost nothing that you are more judgmental and critical about than your body. In a physical practice, criticism and judgment are going to arise, and it becomes an opportunity to stop feeding mental energy and unconscious loyalty to these qualities. And when you practice that, then those qualities start to diminish because it's not getting what it needs to be strong. You notice it, but smile (because you caught yourself) and pull your attention away from it and back to whatever is happening to your life in that moment.

One Size Doesn't Fit All

Vanity and ego are the program we've been spoon-fed by the media since we could open our eyes. We look at a dancer's or athlete's body, toned and cut to shreds, and we say that is healthy—but the truth is that is completely fucked. That has nothing to do with being healthy. These people—dancers puking up their meals and performing injured, athletes taking drugs and abusing their bodies by constantly pushing themselves and dying in their 50s because of how hard they were in their 20s—have nothing to do with health, but we think they epitomize that.

In the pursuit of vanity, we're constantly comparing and competing, not just with others but with ourselves. And it is ridiculous! You can't rationally compare and compete with anyone, including yourself—unless you disrespect yourself—because we are so different and we're always changing. There's nothing more pathetic than comparing and competing, but that's what the rat race is based on. We have catchphrases describing that mentality including "Keeping up with the Joneses." But the Joneses are some seriously messed-up people.

Aging Gracefully

I've always taught what I practice and my rhetoric has reflected that. But the content of my routine and the focus of what I verbally share in class has changed over the years. It's changed because I've changed. I now have two titanium discs in my spine, and I'm not 20 anymore. Routines need to change in order to stay healthful; that's what I practice and it still works. I've simplified what I do in my practice these days, but it's still challenging. At 50, it won't be like I was when I was 20, and at 70, it won't be like 50. The same goes for my teaching: it won't feel authentic if I am not teaching what I am practicing or am just remembering old routines from some time in my history that don't fit the moment.

I remain in the moment and I can acknowledge the change. I wanted to do a handstand push-up in my practice this morning and then realized it wasn't happening and moved on. Years ago, I could have burned through fifteen of them without a problem. But it's not happening now. The strength wasn't there, and there was no judgment or criticism. If there had been judgment, I would have just noticed it, smiled, and moved on. It's aging gracefully. And that's happened because I was taking my own medicine. I am less angry, less vain, less attached to all this shit because yoga works. I still have a long way to go, but I've already gone a long way. What I've achieved inspired me to keep going because

I can see it's working. If it's worked for me, it can work for other people —and it has.

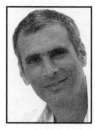

Bryan Kest, who coined the now-ubiquitous term Power Yoga, is a world-renowned international yoga teacher and owner of Santa Monica Power Yoga studios. Bryan is also the creator of donation-based yoga. He has been practicing yoga since 1979, starting when he was 15 years old in Hawaii with David Williams, the first person to bring Ashtanga yoga to America. He also studied in India in 1989 with K. Pattabhi Jois. In addition to teaching locally at his studio in Santa Monica and his international teaching schedule, Bryan allows anyone to practice yoga anywhere with his live-streaming video series at Power Yoga On Demand. www.poweryoga.com

Author photo by kwakualston—kwakualston.com.

DOING MORE BY DOING LESS

Ryan McGraw

At the age of 19, I took my first yoga class. My mom had been asking me to take a yoga class for months. She thought it would be very beneficial for my strength, flexibility, and mental well-being. Having cerebral palsy (CP), doing exercise to keep my strength and flexibility is very important. However, I was convinced that yoga was not for me. After all, I was a male high school senior, and in my mind yoga was a flowery workout that was reserved for women. It was definitely not cool for a teenage guy to do yoga!

The other reason for my apprehension was that I do have CP. Questions ran through my mind: Would I be able to successfully do a yoga class? How would I look in a yoga class? Would I be on display because of my CP? Although these questions were in my head and did play a part in my apprehension, the fact that my masculinity might be questioned by my friends and others was my number one concern.

I finally relented and decided to try a class at our health club to please my mom. I don't remember the poses done in the class, but what I do remember is having a unique, peaceful feeling after *savasana*—that feeling you get after a good yoga practice. This surprised me because all my life I had been an active person. At this time I was swimming six times a week preparing for a competition, but I'd never felt that profoundly peaceful, connected feeling after a workout. I just brushed it off as a "weird feeling," though, and when my mom asked me how I enjoyed class, I simply said it was okay.

I continued to take yoga classes throughout that summer. Most of the classes were with my teacher and friend to this day, Chris. Chris and I connected almost immediately. He made me feel okay about being a man who practiced yoga! Not only this, but he was, and still is, an awesome and inspirational teacher who has a great understanding of yoga.

As time passed, those feelings of apprehension coming from being a male person with CP practicing yoga began to dissipate. They certainly did not completely disappear. I still notice when I am the only male in a yoga class or the class is doing a pose that I cannot perform. Even though I still notice these things, I have become perfectly fine with the fact that I may be in a class with all women or that I may have a different expression of a certain pose than everyone else in the class.

Guys and Yoga?

I must admit, for those first couple of years doing yoga, I was hesitant to let my male friends know I practiced (and *liked*) yoga. When I did let a few friends know, the news was met with a laugh and a condescending comment about my masculinity. Though these comments were made jokingly, they made me self-conscious. The stereotypical image of a young adult male is one of lifting weights in the gym, not doing yoga to soft music in a dimly lit room. It's just not "cool." And certainly not "masculine."

I have invited a few of those same friends to take yoga with me over the years. They have been humbled by the physicality of the workout. They have commented, "My muscles are so tight," "That was a tough workout," and "I need to do this more." Their perception of yoga changed after they took a class. I think with yoga's growing popularity, and with the advent of new styles of fitness-based yoga over the past ten years, it has become more culturally acceptable for men to do yoga. However, I don't know if the perception of yoga among males in high school and young adulthood has changed. There is a lot of peer pressure at that age and a lot of emphasis on fitting in. I became more comfortable with the fact that I was a male doing yoga as I matured. As I matured, the people around me matured too, and yoga just became something that I did.

Over the next two years, I took classes here and there primarily for my physical benefit. During this time I understood how yoga could benefit me physically. My goal was to do the full expression of every pose. For example, I wanted to touch the floor in *trikonasana* (Triangle pose) or keep up with the class when they were doing Sun Salutations quickly. I wanted to do poses and go for poses like everyone else in the class, not understanding the potential risk of injury that put me at. For example, one may be able to touch the ground in *trikonasana*, but if they are dumping into their low back, totally out of alignment, unsteady and not breathing properly, they are putting themselves at a great risk of injury. Thus, at this point in my yoga journey I did not understand the principles of adaptation and the positive benefits of modification as they related to my body.

Custom Yoga

During my sophomore year of college, I became increasingly interested in yoga for its therapeutic benefits. One night I decided to take a class at a yoga studio that had just opened up. It was a level 2/3 class, but I figured I could handle it. I had met the teacher of the class, Karina Mirsky, briefly in the past, so I thought it would be no problem. It was a problem, though!

Karina thought it would be in my best interest if I came back for a level 1 or level ½ class. However, I managed to convince her that I would be okay. During the class it became clear that the question was not whether I could do the poses (I did the poses in the way I was used to doing them), but whether I could do the poses in a safe manner. Karina did what she could to keep me safe in the class by adjusting me. She saw that I risked injury in various poses because my body was out of alignment. I needed to find a way to adapt or modify some of the yoga poses.

After class we talked and decided that I should do a private session. I did not really know what to expect in a private session with her, but I knew she had worked with individuals with disabilities before with both yoga and massage.

When we began the session, Karina announced that we would begin our practice in a chair. I thought this was interesting, as I had never practiced yoga seated in a chair before, but I was more than willing to give it a try. We did a few poses in the chair: arm raises, a twist, a seated forward fold, and probably a few more I don't remember.

What was stressed throughout that session was the importance of adapting poses for my own individual needs. I did not need to go for the full expression of every pose because doing so could be harmful. I needed to discover the expression of the pose that suited *my* body. When I adapted poses to the needs of my body, my body was in better alignment. As a result, I am still getting the benefits of the pose even though the form of the pose may be different from the other bodies in class.

Since I have spastic cerebral palsy and my entire body is affected, there are a variety of adaptations/modifications I do. Even though I do not adapt every yoga pose, I probably could! The poses that I need to adapt/modify the most are standing poses, because I am often off balance in these poses. When I am off balance, I activate the wrong muscles to get into poses, thus putting unnecessary stress on my body and not finding ease in the pose. An example of an adaptation I do is Triangle pose with my back against the wall, bringing my hand to the back of a chair. Of course, standing poses are not the only ones I adapt. Since my lower back rounds when I do seated poses, I always sit on a blanket (which is a very common adaptation that is encouraged in many yoga classes). The complexity of the adaptation I choose often depends on the pace of class I am in, but I always try to keep my body safe in poses.

Though I did not buy in totally to this philosophy after a single yoga session, something had clicked. I began to work with Karina more and apply these principles of adaptation to regular yoga classes that I took, becoming more concerned with setting up poses properly than attempting to keep up with the class. I became more enthusiastic about yoga and wanted to gain as much knowledge I could about this discipline by taking workshops and interning at my friend Chris's yoga studio the summers of my sophomore and junior year of college.

More Layers

As my physical practice of the *asanas* began to become my own, I found that the mental and spiritual aspects of my practice started to fall into place. I attribute this to the fact that by respecting the needs of my body instead of struggling in poses, I was able to focus on other things within the pose. I could become aware of my breath, which is the foundation of yoga poses. With the breath I was able to go deeper into my practice, through the breath and respecting the needs of my body.

Through combining breath and movement, I was better able to feel a calmness when I practiced. But to really be able to focus on the breath when I practice, I need to respect the needs of my body. For example, if I am doing a standing forward fold, I can touch the ground. However, I would most likely not have a consistent breath and would not be doing the pose in alignment. If I brought my hands to a chair or blocks, I would much more likely be connected with my breath and have a more consistent breath. Alignment of the body enhances the quality of breath, which in turn enhances the quality of mind. The connection of all three is vital to yoga.

In 2008, I moved to Chicago to begin graduate school and found a number of great yoga teachers in the first few months. One day after class, the teacher asked me if I had ever been to the gentle class at the Yoga Circle. I had heard of this class from a friend but had never attended. The class sounded very interesting and exactly what I was looking for since it stressed the adaptation of poses. It was a class in which an apprentice of the teacher Gabriel Halpern worked with you one to one. It was not a private or a special yoga therapy class; it was just another yoga class on the schedule.

One day in the winter of 2009, I decided to give the class a try. The Yoga Circle is an Iyengar yoga studio. Iyengar yoga is a style of yoga that is based upon precise anatomical alignment. As I walked into the studio, I was shocked by the amount of props they had. Not only did the studio have the basic yoga props such as blankets, bolsters, blocks, and straps, but it had *many* others—all with the purpose to get the yoga practitioner in the form of the pose that's right for their body. I remember feeling a little like a beginner in that first class because Gabriel wanted me to do basic poses. In my mind, I was an experienced yoga practitioner, practicing yoga for six years before coming that day. After class I asked Gabriel what other classes on the schedule would suit my needs. He recommended that I just do the gentle class for now until I learned more about how to adapt the poses for my body. This hurt my ego since I had been practicing for years and had modified poses to the extent I needed to benefit my body, or at least I thought I had.

Although my ego was bruised and I did not stop going to other yoga classes, I started going to the Yoga Circle on a weekly basis. There I learned how to adapt my poses on a whole new level, a level that required me to be more observant of the needs of my body. The props were there to support me, and I was encouraged to use them as needed to maximize the integrity of my yoga practice. I found a better understanding of my body. Let me give you an example to better explain what I mean. In *supta padangusthasana* (a supine hamstring stretch) one leg is lifted straight up in the air and the other is extended straight out on the ground. If you cannot reach the toe of the foot that is extended in the air, you can loop a belt around the foot and hold both ends of the belt. This would be the adaptation encouraged in most yoga classes. However, Iyengar yoga takes the adaptation further so that the practitioner is supported. The way I would do this pose is lying down with my feet pressing against a wall. The back of my grounded leg is supported by a folded blanket since it does not reach the ground, and I place a block against the wall so I can really press through the foot. Then I loop a belt around the other foot and raise that leg only to point where I can still keep it straight.

This kind of attention to detail made my practice stronger. I felt more integrated within my body with the emphasis on alignment and creating a stronger mind-body connection. Not only was I gaining greater body awareness, but I was gaining greater mental awareness of my practice and other areas of life off the yoga mat.

Sharing Yoga with Others

From the time I discovered how to use adaptation, I wanted to take yoga teacher training and bring adaptive yoga to others. Until I came to Yoga Circle, I didn't feel I was ready to delve into a teacher training, even though I had attended many workshops with master teachers and had taken a portion of a teacher training for my own knowledge. It was all of my combined experiences in yoga that gave me the confidence to finally make the commitment. I know that anyone can do a yoga teacher training, but to me it was very important to have a strong practice and understand yoga on and off the mat.

Another thing that contributed to my decision to take teacher training and bring my knowledge of yoga to students was reading *Waking: A Memoir of Trauma and Transcendence*, by Matthew Sanford. Matthew sustained a spinal cord injury when he was in a car accident at age 13. While he was in traditional rehabilitation, doctors and therapists told him to focus on regaining strength in his upper body and that he would never regain control in his lower body. Thus, the medical field told him to ignore his lower body.

Matthew went through life feeling like there was always something missing. He believed that control of his lower limbs was possible, but he did not know how to access this control—that is, until he discovered yoga. Through yoga, Matthew was able to establish a mind-body connection and once again have a fully integrated body. This is something that I can relate to in my own body, moving through yoga in a way that I never experienced before. Matthew went on to become an Iyengar yoga teacher and create Mind Body Solutions, a nonprofit organization whose mission is to awaken the connection between the mind and body.

Even though I knew that yoga could benefit everyone, there was a part of me that questioned if I could become a certified yoga teacher as a person with a disability. How would I demonstrate the correct form of yoga poses? How would I adjust students? How would I keep students safe?

The answer to how I would teach was really quite simple and was staring me in the face all along: I would adapt teaching to my abilities.

The goal is still to give students the best experience possible, but I have to respect my abilities while doing it. This may mean I teach seated yoga or use words to adjust students rather than touch. If I'm teaching an adaptive yoga class to people of different abilities, I have assistants to help students get into the yoga poses. My goal when teaching is not to impress students by doing an advanced form of a yoga pose; instead, my goal is to get them into a pose safely and correctly so they are able to receive the benefits of the pose.

The teacher training that I took at Prairie Yoga was exactly what I was looking for. It encouraged adaptation, proper alignment, and great overall teaching skills. I felt as if it gave me a solid foundation to teach students and taught me a great deal about my own practice.

Teacher training is just one step in my yoga journey and there is still much left to learn as a yoga practitioner. My collective yoga experience is what got me to where I am today. The only way I am going to be a successful yoga teacher and student, especially with adaptive yoga, is to continue learning. Everyone has a unique body, thus there is no single adaptation of a pose that fits all. Each yoga practitioner needs to practice yoga based on their ability, remembering there is no right or wrong expression of yoga.

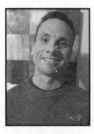

Ryan McGraw is a yoga teacher and advocate for people with disabilities. He also holds a master's degree in disability and human development. As a person with a disability himself, Ryan believes that yoga can be made accessible and be adapted for people of all abilities. He feels that everyone should be able to receive the benefits of yoga.

Author photo by Karen McGraw.

VIRABHADRASANA IN THE ACADEMY: COMING OUT WITH AN OPEN HEART

Dr. Audrey Bilger

Warrior I

Step forward, bend front knee, raise arms overhead,
gaze up, and lift your heart.

Lesbian Counteroffensive. As I read this phrase on a piece of paper I found in my mailbox at school, I felt a shock run through my body. I looked around the faculty support center and could see that this page had been placed in all the cubbyholes. Upon closer examination, I understood exactly what it meant. I was the lesbian, and this was war.

I have been teaching English and gender studies at a small private college in southern California since the mid-1990s, and when, in the spring of 2001, I discovered what turned out to be a leaked conspiracy memo in the mailroom, at first I thought it was more of the usual brand of campus intrigue: conservatives versus liberals, traditionalists versus multiculturalists. Turns out, this document was a strategic battle plan drafted by an anonymous cadre of right-wing professors: a to-do list for undermining the college's recently installed president and dean, who were perceived by those formerly in power as progressive and hence a threat to the status quo. The bullet-pointed memo included the names of influential donors to contact, along with other actions that, if accomplished, would almost certainly have toppled the new regime. Whoever typed up the document had left it in a copy machine, and some other individual had decided to shine a spotlight on this nefarious plot by making photocopies for the entire faculty.

When most people think about academia, they probably imagine a bucolic realm of absentminded scholars and hushed library aisles. Even though the widely recognized phrase "publish or perish" hints at the potential for hostility and strife, nonacademics know little about the abuses that frequently occur within the so-called ivory tower.

The Bigger the Sharks

My wife and I often joke about how, as rough as her male-dominated work world is—she's in the music business—the academy can be even more brutal. The smaller the fish tank, the bigger the sharks.

As soon as I saw that some sort of lesbian "counteroffensive" was in the works, I knew I was the only possible target. My school skewed conservative at that time, so much so that before I was tenured, I was advised not to come out as a lesbian. Once I got tenure and made my way out of the closet, I became a resource for a number of gay male students who sought to reconcile their sexual orientation with this confining environment; however, in spite of my visibility, I didn't know a single other lesbian on campus.

My conservative colleagues clearly felt threatened by me. Why else would they have proposed a *counter* attack? In military terms, a counteroffensive is, after all, a response to a prior action by an enemy force. What I realized as I stood in the mailroom staring at the evidence of their animosity was that I was exposed. I had been singled out, not because of the quality of my work, but because I dared to be open about my identity. My very being was deemed "offensive," and my body bore the initial blow. I braced myself for a possible attack. I froze—clenched jaw, tight shoulders, and rigid spine.

Braced for Battle

Because the climate on my campus had already been chilly for me from the beginning of my time there—the faculty had only a handful of women then—I always tensed up when I walked on campus. Early on, I stopped wearing skirts and tended to dress in dark colors, even though I love clothes, and left to my own devices, I'm happy to wear color, pattern, and ornamentation. In the classroom and in meetings, I could tell that female bodies did not carry authority in this community. After I came out as gay, I began to be even more conscious of my body on campus. I certainly did not belong to anybody's old boys' network. I was something queer and other. Camouflage was strategic. I thought I could *be* out, and even *speak* out, but not necessarily *stand* out. Those who knew could know, and those who didn't would, I thought, leave me in peace.

To complicate matters even further, when I first started teaching here, I had arrived with a husband in tow, who became an ex-husband shortly thereafter when I came out to myself and identified as a lesbian. When you go from being straight to gay, your physical body doesn't change. You look in the mirror into the same eyes you've always known. You have the same skin color, height, vital statistics, and shoe size. You might choose to get piercings and tattoos; you might adopt a wardrobe that announces your queerness to the world; or you might, as I did, simply go on with your life and not display in any outward way the metamorphosis that had taken place. Having lived more than thirty years as a straight woman, I was unaware of my own heterosexual privilege until I lost it. I never imagined I would have to arm myself for warfare.

Admittedly, the battles that came to me were minor when compared to those faced by abandoned queer kids on the streets, lesbians and gays in countries that imprison homosexuals, or anyone in the midst of actual, violent wars. The metaphor of warfare was thrust upon me by my militaristic colleagues, who were engaged in the culture wars with me in their crosshairs, and I felt their malice seep into my bloodstream. Walking onto campus required a daily dose of courage.

The lesbian counteroffensive memo forced me into the trenches. I grew fearful—for my personal safety and for my career. I distrusted almost everyone I encountered. I looked over my shoulder. I even considered leaving this job that I had worked so hard to get. Fight or flight—those seemed to be the choices.

Meeting the Warrior

As the drama unfolded, I found solace in my long-established yoga practice. Each morning I would unroll my mat, quiet my breath, and move into a state of equilibrium. I first discovered the healing power of yoga when I was a graduate student, suffering from back pain and headaches. From the very beginning, my practice brought balance and stability to my world. Rather than tensing up in the midst of struggle, I learned to breathe into challenges—inhalations for strength, exhalations for flexibility. Yoga did more than just eliminate my physical ailments; it improved the quality of my academic work and my life.

Because I am a literary scholar and writer, I have always particularly loved the metaphorical aspects of yoga. In Mountain pose, my feet become grounded and my mind expands into the heavens; in child's pose, I fold into myself and feel safe and protected. It makes sense that ultimately the metaphors of yoga enacted daily on the mat brought me solace when forces at my school conspired to do battle with me. I came to see my situation more clearly in my daily practice, and I understood that I would not have to engage in an endless struggle nor would I have to flee. Instead, I could be a warrior and move through the challenges with grace and dignity, continually renewing my energy and staying the course. I would take the warrior path and endure.

Warrior II

Step to the side, point right toe outward, bend knee, spread arms wide,
turn your head to gaze over right arm, and lift your heart.

D-Day

Once the lesbian counteroffensive memo became public, as part of what was clearly a plan to fracture the college, the faculty was up in arms. The administration called a special meeting, and I counted the hours as the date approached with dread. I knew that no matter how the discussion proceeded, I would be in the spotlight.

I couldn't sleep the night before. Adrenaline coursed through my veins. I had a pretty clear idea which of my "colleagues" were behind the memo, and their faces kept appearing before me. I imagined confronting them directly. I wanted to see them punished. A few hours before sunrise, I climbed out of bed, stumbling in the half-light to my study. I turned on the computer and opened a file.

I decided I would confront my antagonists at this meeting. I had nowhere to hide, and I no longer wanted to. Because I knew it would be impossible for me to stay calm and say what needed to be said, I wrote a speech. I typed furiously, expressing the pain of having been closeted, describing the contemptuous looks from anti-gay individuals that seared their way into my skin, sharing stories about gay students who came to me to share their sorrow and frustration. The lesbian counteroffensive, I would say at the end, was an affront not just to me but also to the aspirations of higher education, and I expressed my belief that our community could do better.

At first, my wife tried to talk me out of speaking. She was anxious, but as she would later explain, she recognized the look on my face as one of resolve and certitude. She held me close and told me she was proud of me.

Before I left the house, I called a gay male friend, who was familiar with the politics of my campus, and told him what I planned to say.

"You'll be so alone," he fretted.

After I hung up, I thought about that point. I already felt alone. How could speaking out make me feel any more isolated? I wanted to be heard and understood. In the car on my drive to school, an idea came to me, and I mentally added another step to my plan.

The Moment of Truth

When I entered the large lecture hall where the meeting was being held, I braced myself for what might happen. Was everyone staring at me or did I just feel on display? My eyes sought out the people I believed were responsible for the plot. There were probably five or six in the group, I guessed. All present. I didn't want to tremble, but I couldn't help it.

What became clear right away was that the memo writers would not be "outed" at this meeting. Representatives of the administration spoke about investigations underway and about possible legal problems arising from the memo. I clutched the printout in my hands, waiting for an opportunity to step forward.

As soon as the floor was opened for comments, I made my way to the front. I had deliberately taken a seat near the podium. Still, my steps were unsteady, and my knees quaked. I delivered my remarks as forcefully as I could, looking up occasionally yet unable to gauge the reaction from my audience.

After I concluded my prepared statement, I turned my full attention to the room and took stock. I wanted to avoid experiencing the isolation my friend feared would be my lot.

"Now I need to know who stands with me in deploring the bigotry of this memo," I announced. "I want to see a show of hands."

I looked around and saw that a few people were shifting in their seats uncomfortably, but others looked receptive and encouraging.

One person shouted, "What are we voting on? Is this an official vote?"

I stood my ground. "I just need to know who I'm working with. Raise your hands if you join me in denouncing the memo and if you support a welcoming climate for LGBT people."

Much to my surprise, virtually everyone—even those I knew to be responsible for the memo (covering their backs, no doubt)—put a hand in the air. I had almost unanimous support.

I went back to my seat and somehow made it through the rest of the meeting without collapsing. Over the next few days, my e-mail inbox filled with messages of solidarity, both from people I knew well and from those I had barely ever spoken to. Later that year, I received a distinguished merit award, voted on by the entire faculty.

Embodying the Warrior

In spite of the many indications of support I received, this incident took its toll. I felt increasingly weary and burned out. The memo writers were never named or publicly shamed. I saw them in the halls and in faculty meetings. Although the climate showed some signs of improvement, I continued to hear stories from students about their sense of alienation and anxiety. I kept up my yoga practice and benefited from the regular infusions of calm I found there, but I had yet to grasp the warrior's lesson.

Warrior III

Raise arms over head, gaze up, step forward; bending from the waist,
extend your back leg off the ground and bring your torso parallel
to the ground, eyes ahead, heart lifted.

A couple of years after combating the lesbian counteroffensive, I was in a yoga class. As the teacher encouraged us to let go into a forward fold, I suddenly realized there was so much I wanted to release. I thought about my school and how I disliked spending time there. I harbored anger and residual fear. I was expected to go up for another promotion, but I resisted putting myself at the mercy of the bullies in whose eyes I felt constantly judged and found wanting.

The negativity that made my body tense up at work was not specific to me as an out lesbian. Academic culture is all about grades, evaluation, and assessment. To get a professorship, you have to spend years in graduate school and complete a PhD, then undergo job searches where you're up against a hundred or more candidates. You must submit articles and books for publication and face review committees at every turn. It's a veritable judgment wheel.

Yoga practitioners have long understood the value of being wholehearted. In the Warrior sequence and in backbends, we celebrate the heart's courage, and we cultivate balance and centeredness in the midst of life's relentless upheavals.

On the mat that morning in yoga class, I followed my instructor's guidance and exhaled into the pose, relaxing muscles whose tension I hadn't even noticed a moment ago as I consciously released the burden I'd been carrying. I felt my heart engage and my senses clear.

I saw then that if I wanted to thrive in my work rather than continue to absorb the stress in my body and exist in survival mode, I needed to open my heart. In all the time I had been practicing yoga, I had considered the Warrior sequence from an embattled perspective. Life is a struggle, I had thought. Yoga will provide a refuge, a barricade, a place of protection.

Standing upright once again after the forward fold and preparing to step into *Virabhadrasana*, I felt absolutely light and present. My heart expanded, like that cartoon of the Grinch who reforms his Christmas-thwarting ways when he releases anger and makes room for love.

Fierce

Warrior pose, I came to see, is about allowing yourself be vulnerable, fiercely offering your heart to the world, and braving the possibility—the near certainty, even—of rejection, judgment, hostility. In the purest moment of the here and now, there is no struggle. Balance, grace, open-heartedness—these are the yogic warrior's tools. With this insight, I could move forward.

I spent the next summer completing a yoga teacher training program near where I lived. I spoke to the athletics program at my school and asked whether, in addition to my academic offerings, I could teach a PE class in the fall. I brought my practice to campus, and in the process, I began to humanize my workplace, forge new ties with my colleagues and coworkers, and engage in a different form of connection with my students.

Ten years after incorporating yoga into my academic environment, I no longer tense up when I walk on campus. Instead, I straighten my shoulders, lift my head, and offer my heart. There is no separation between what I do on the mat and my orientation in the classroom, the contentious faculty meeting, or a trip to the beach, for that matter. In each instance, I try to center my awareness and embrace vulnerability.

Being openly gay is just one version of being authentic and true to oneself in an environment that might not accept your truth. What gay rights history has shown is that being in the closet—hiding your authentic self—will not protect you. When I spoke out and asked my colleagues to connect with me, I was, in effect, teaching my first yoga class at my college. The lesbian counteroffensive—whatever that was—dissolved, or if it continued, it did so in secrecy and public silence.

Colleagues tell me I paved the way for additional positive changes. Some even say they view me as a role model. I know that changing my posture from defensive, embattled fighter to open-hearted yogic warrior made academic life better for me, and I'm overjoyed to think that I help to make this life better for others.

These days I measure my accomplishments in terms of connections. I combat the tendency in the academy to be always comparing and criticizing. Battle lines can be barriers to self-discovery, and on my ever-evolving path, I strive to see myself in those who might call me the enemy.

Like a true warrior, I step forward, find balance, and open my heart.

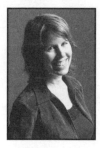

Audrey Bilger, PhD, is the faculty director of the Center for Writing and Public Discourse and professor of literature and gender studies at Claremont McKenna College. Her most recent book, which she coedited with Michele Kort, is *Here Come the Brides! Reflections on Lesbian Love and Marriage.* She is the author of *Laughing Feminism: Subversive Comedy in Frances Burney, Maria Edgeworth, and Jane Austen* and editor of Jane Collier's 1753 *Essay on the Art of Ingeniously Tormenting* for Broadview Literary Texts. Her work has appeared in *Ms.* magazine, the *Ms.* blog, *Bitch* magazine, the *Los Angeles Times*, and she is the gender/sexuality editor of the *Los Angeles Review of Books.*

Author photo by Greg Allen.

WHERE WE GO FROM HERE

Anna Guest-Jelley

Wow, right?

If you're like us, your head is spinning with insights, connections, and ways to move forward from here. We're grateful to each of our amazing writers for sharing their stories with such courage, vulnerability, and wisdom.

We know that now is the time to expand this conversation. Our hope is that this book will be a springboard into conversations in local communities about how yoga can be a tool for supporting body image, and how current yoga students and teachers can challenge each other in helpful ways to make their yoga spaces places where everyone is welcomed as they are.

This does not mean, as we saw in the essays, asking people who are currently on the margins on yoga, or not even currently practicing, to "fit in" with yoga-culture-as-usual. Rather, it's a call to change yoga-culture-as-usual.

Fortunately, we have a model for this: the practice of yoga, which draws us into deeper connection with our own body and wisdom, as well as into *sangha*, or community. The ethical precepts of yoga, the *yamas* and *niyamas*, have much to teach us about how to pave a way forward. From the compassion of *ahimsa* to the self-study of *svadhyaya*, the practice challenges us to work toward more union—with mind, body, and each other.

How to Work with Your Body Image through Yoga

As these essays have shown, although yoga's relationship with body image is complex, it is possible to work with your own through yoga.

We believe this is best done with the support of a wise and thoughtful yoga teacher, as well as whatever other support is helpful for you, possibly including a doctor, therapist, and/or nutritionist. It's important to know that while yoga can be an incredible tool for healing your body image, it doesn't exist in a vacuum and should be considered one tool in a toolbox of various types of support.

We believe, our essays have shown, and research supports the idea that the way yoga helps people with their body image is because of how it connects people with their body. After all, it's hard to improve how you feel about your body when you don't actually know how you feel *in* your body.

When yoga teachers ask you to do something like "Feel your back leg in Warrior I," that may feel a bit esoteric to people who have a history of disconnection with their body. But given time, that instruction becomes less metaphorical and more concrete.

This is especially true when it's specifically guided, whether in a group class or your home practice. For example, here's one way you might experiment with this on your own:

1. Come into Down Dog (in the traditional version on the floor, or in a modified version with your hands on a stable chair seat).

2. Take five deep breaths here and notice how you're feeling in this moment—particularly check in with your hips and shoulders, making a mental note of where they feel less open than you might like. File this info away because you'll be coming back to it.

3. Do three of your favorite, gentle hip-opening poses. Some you might consider include a lunge pose (standing or kneeling), Pigeon pose (with or without the support of a blanket), and a standing wide-legged forward bend.

4. Come back to Down Dog, doing it the same way you did the first time. Again, take five deep breaths and notice how you're feeling. Check in with your hips and shoulders, noting any differences from the first time you did the pose.

5. Do three of your favorite, gentle shoulder-opening poses. Some you might consider include Cow-Faced pose (with a strap), slow shoulder rolls, and a Wall Clock.

6. Come back to Down Dog, doing it the same way as you did the first two times. For the last time in this position, take five deep breaths. While you're here, check in with how you feel, and note any differences in your hips and shoulders.

7. Come back to standing and continue with your day.

You can always add on to the practice above or try it with a different pose. Whatever you do, the intention remains the same: to return to the same pose multiple times throughout a practice in order to notice whatever shifts might arise in your body as you go along.

Practices such as these can be key for helping rebuild a clear connection between mind and body and build the ability to know and notice what is going on in your body.

Recommendations for Teachers

While yoga practitioners can use yoga as a tool to improve their body image on their own, they also need the support of thoughtful and skillful teachers, particularly when practicing in group classes. When teachers create a body-positive environment in their classes, it makes space for people to practice what we think yoga is all about—connecting with your own mind and body, exactly as they are in this moment.

Some people argue that creating a body-positive environment allows people to opt out of caring for themselves. But we think the opposite is true: it's only when you accept yourself as you are that you're able to take loving action to feel your best.

Here are some ways that yoga teachers can bring more body positivity into their classes:

Room setup

When possible, consider asking students to set up with the short end of their mat to the wall. Not only does this give people easy access to the wall for poses (hello, balancing poses and getting up/down off the floor with a little more grace!), it also allows everyone to see and hear a little better because they don't have their neighbor's foot (on a good day) in their face.

Ask open-ended questions

Want to support each student in a way that works for them? First, you have to know them. Rather than asking a yes/no question ("Do you have any injuries?"), consider an open-ended question ("Tell me about what's going on with your body"). This approach both gives you more information and gives you a moment to build connection and rapport with the student.

Work from most supported to least supported

Many yoga classes start by teaching the least supported version of the pose (e.g., *trikonasana*, Triangle pose with hand to the floor) and then offer options "if you can't do it" (e.g., a block under the bottom hand). To make your classes more empowering for everyone, consider doing the reverse. Start everyone with a block under the hand and build confidence and strength. Then, if/when students are feeling stable, offer suggestions for lowering or removing the block—making lots of space, of course, for people to not do that.

Talk about It

Have regular conversations with your students, both during and before/after class, about your class being a space to greet their body exactly as it is. You can also weave body-positive themes into your classes to deepen the experience.

The other thing teachers can do is consider how their own body image is affecting their teaching. For example, if a teacher doesn't feel good about their body, that will often get projected onto the class with comments about "working off a muffin top" or other comments along those lines.

As a teacher, you don't have to have a perfect body image to create a supportive environment for your students. Not even close (because we're pretty sure such a thing doesn't even exist anyway). What you can do instead, though, is do your own work on your body image, just like you are inviting your students to do. When you raise your consciousness about the language you use about your own body, it raises your awareness about what you might be sharing with your students.

Improving body image is an ongoing process for all of us, and the best way teachers can show up for their students is by being honest about that and being willing to be on the path with them.

Resources

Want support around navigating yoga, body image, or how they intersect? We have you covered with some of these great organizations:

National Eating Disorders Association

Resources and local eating disorder support (US only).
www.nationaleatingdisorders.org

The Art of Yoga Project

Yoga and art for incarcerated teen girls.
www.theartofyogaproject.org

Adios Barbie

Body image and body-positive resources.
www.adiosbarbie.com

Proud2BMe

Body image for teens.
www.proud2bme.org

And, of course, check out the author bios following each essay to visit the websites of our contributors. Each of them is doing work around this issue in their own way, and they have many helpful resources to offer!

Keep in Touch

We're excited to see where this conversation goes—for individuals, yoga teachers, yoga communities, and beyond.

We'd love to stay in touch and hear about how the book has affected you. Connect with us online at www.yogaandbodyimage.com, like us on Facebook (www.facebook.com/YogaAndBodyImage), and follow us on Twitter (@YogaBodyImage).

Acknowledgments

We'd like to thank all of our contributors for bravely sharing their stories with such honesty, vulnerability, and beauty. You have touched us deeply and inspire us with your courage and wisdom. We are so very grateful for each of you.

We want to give special acknowledgment to Vytas Baskauskas, Ruby Corley, Seane Corn, Angela Wix and the team at Llewellyn, Elyse Tanzillo, and Frank Weiman. Without you, this book would not be the special collection of voices that it is.

We also want to thank the teachers who have taught and inspired us over the years. In addition, we want to acknowledge our wonderful students who compel us to continue doing this work. You are also our teachers and a beacon of light.

Finally, we want to express our love and appreciation for the family and friends who buoy us daily. You make all our efforts worth it. We love you.

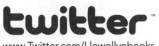

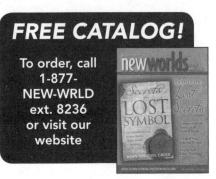

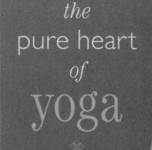

the
pure heart
of
yoga

Ten Essential Steps for
Personal Transformation

Robert Butera, Ph.D.

The Pure Heart of Yoga
Ten Essential Steps for Personal Transformation
ROBERT BUTERA PHD

Connect to the infinite through yoga and experience true transformation on the physical, emotional, psychological, and spiritual planes.

This inspiring book teaches yoga the way the original masters envisioned it—a holistic union of body, mind, and spirit. Dr. Butera's simple ten-step approach invites all levels of yoga practitioners and teachers to deepen their understanding of yoga philosophy and work toward health and self-realization. By cultivating a mindful practice of the yoga postures, you will learn to balance emotions, focus the mind, control breathing, work with the body's energy centers (chakras), eliminate psychological blocks, and create a sense of purpose and peace for life.

978-0-7387-1487-5, 336 pp., 6 x 9   **$21.95**

The Yoga of Food

of

Food

Wellness from the Inside Out

Healing the
Relationship with
Food & Your
Body

Melissa Grabau, PhD

The Yoga of Food
Wellness from the Inside Out
MELISSA GRABAU PHD

For the millions of people who struggle with food and body issues, yoga and its practice of mindfulness can offer a surprisingly effective path to well-being. For Melissa Grabau, a psychotherapist who has battled her own eating disorders since she was a child, yoga contains the key ingredients to transforming our connection to food and to our bodies.

The Yoga of Food invites you to explore contemplation prompts and meditations that will help you create a deeper appreciation of the body's health and vitality. Sharing lessons and stories she's cultivated from years of clinical practice, Melissa provides a roadmap toward a healthier approach to nutrition and the human spirit.

978-0-7387-4015-7, 264 pp., 6 x 9   **$16.99**

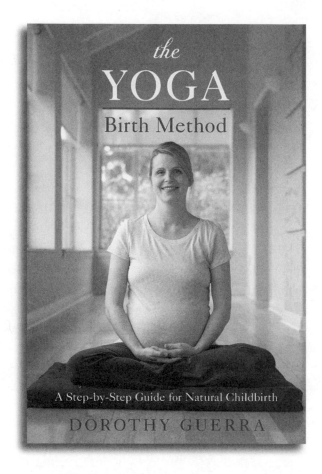

the

YOGA

Birth Method

A Step-by-Step Guide for Natural Childbirth

DOROTHY GUERRA

The Yoga Birth Method
A Step-by-Step Guide for Natural Childbirth
DOROTHY GUERRA

Plan a childbirth that's calm, natural, and enlightened. *The Yoga Birth Method* is an empowering eight-step pathway to achieving a positive and joyful birth experience.

Applying the wisdom of yoga to childbirth, Dorothy Guerra offers a solid plan for managing the mind, body, and spirit throughout the stages of pregnancy and labor. Couples choose an intention that becomes a focal point for embracing a calm state of mind throughout the physical and emotional challenges of childbirth. You'll discover what to expect during each stage of labor and how to manage pain, eliminate anxiety, and encourage labor progression with breathing techniques and yoga poses. There's also guidance in drafting a birth plan, labor-support techniques for birth partners, information on medical intervention, and a "go to" chapter with checklists to use when the big day arrives!

978-0-7387-3665-5, 240 pp., 6 x 9 **$15.99**

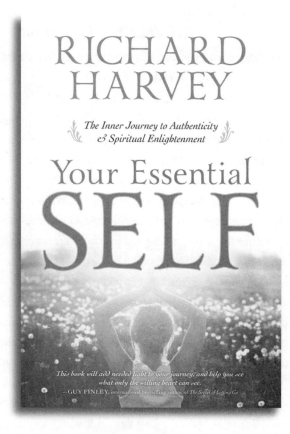

RICHARD
HARVEY

*The Inner Journey to Authenticity
& Spiritual Enlightenment*

Your Essential

SELF

*This book will add needed light to your journey, and help you see
what only the willing heart can see.*
—GUY FINLEY, international bestselling author of *The Secret of Letting Go*

Your Essential Self

The Inner Journey to Authenticity & Spiritual Enlightenment

RICHARD HARVEY

Despite the relationships, possessions, and prestige we all strive for, most people live at only a fraction of their full potential. But with the guidance and wisdom in *Your Essential Self,* you will awaken to your divine nature. Learn how to attain the three stages of human awakening—the process of self-discovery, the transformation into authenticity, and the source of consciousness—on the inner journey to your true self.

This comprehensive guide describes how spiritual attainment is not an unreachable fantasy, but rather a logical extension of human development. The personality, the authentic self, and the transcendent self are discovered through stories from Richard's personal experience, case studies from his therapy practice, questionnaires, and exercises designed for your journey toward self-realization.

978-0-7387-3470-5, 288 pp., 6 x 9 **$15.99**
